PART I FFARCS PRACTICE E[X

PART I FFARCS PRACTICE EXAMS

Wynne Aveling MA MB BChir FFARCS
The Middlesex Hospital, London.

Stuart Ingram MBBS FFARCS
University College Hospital, London.

© 1986 PASTEST SERVICE
304 Galley Hill
Hemel Hempstead, Hertfordshire.
Tel: 0442 52113

All rights reserved. No part of this publication may be reproduced, stored in a retrieval system, or transmitted, in any form or by any means, electronic, mechanical, photocopying, recording or otherwise without the prior permission of the copyright owner.

British Library Cataloguing in Publication Data

Aveling, W.
Practice exams for Part I FFARCS MCQ's,
written paper, case histories and illustrations
1. Anesthesia — Problems, exercises, etc.
I. Title   II. Ingram, S.
617'.96'076   RD82.3

ISBN 0-906896-26-6

Text prepared by Turner Associates, Knutsford, Cheshire.
Phototypeset by Communitype, Leicester.
Printed by Oxford University Press.

CONTENTS

Preface	vii
How to use this book	ix
The Part I FFARCS Examination	1
The Multiple Choice Paper: Introduction	4
How to use the MCQ Papers in this book	7
MCQ Practice Exam 1	9
MCQ Practice Exam 2	24
The Written Paper: Introduction	39
Written Paper 1	41
Written Paper 2	42
Written Paper 3	43
The Orals: Introduction	44
13 Clinical Case Histories with related questions	47
Illustrations	63
Answers and Teaching Explanations	87
MCQ Practice Exam 1	87
MCQ Practice Exam 2	105
Written Paper 1: Outline Answers	124
Written Paper 2: Outline Answers	129
Written Paper 3: Outline Answers	135
Clinical Case History Answers	141
Reading and Reference Books	156
	156
Index	157

PREFACE

When the moment finally comes and the numbers are called out, some will step forward to hear that they have passed. They will head for the pub to enjoy the well earned glow of self-confidence that is induced by a gin and tonic, safe in the knowledge that another exam is safely behind them. But at the other end of the bar there will gather those whose numbers were not called, in all probability they will have worked and studied just as hard and may well know just as much, but as they stare balefully into their mug of bitter they know that they will be back again in a few months for another go.

What made the difference? Some will say luck, or perhaps it was the misfortune of encountering for the Orals one of those examiners so notorious, that in the waiting room their name is not even mentioned in hushed whispers. The real answer is probably much simpler and can be summarised as "organisation and presentation", otherwise referred to as examination technique. The candidate who passed appreciated that the exam is not just about what you have learnt but it is about the ability to recall and relay what you have learnt.

The object of this book is to help those preparing for the exam to achieve that ability and thus to ensure that the publicans sell rather more gin and tonic and rather less bitter.

The idea of writing this book came from our association with others, in setting up and running the North London Course for the Part 1 exam. This course started in the autumn of 1984 and we believe that it has shown that although one of the original intentions of changing the format of the FFA exams was to encourage teaching by consultants of the SHOs in their own hospitals, this often needs to be supplemented. In addition it is vital to know exactly how the exam is being conducted and to talk at length with candidates both successful and unsuccessful to learn how teaching should be modified to improve the chances of success. We are grateful to many of the students on the North London Course who have helped with this feedback and have acted as guinea pigs in the selection of much of the material included here. We would also wish to acknowledge the help of our many clinical colleagues who have provided material for inclusion in this book.

Consultants can sit in at the orals and see both the way in which questions are being asked and also where the candidates show weaknesses in answering. You should urge any consultant interested in teaching to take up this opportunity to sit in. The Faculty of Anaesthetists publishes information about the format of their exams and anyone planning to take an exam should write at an early stage for this information. We have with the Faculty's permission quoted where relevant from this information and in general it has been placed between quotation marks.

HOW TO USE THIS BOOK

There are sections to help with each aspect of the exam, providing general advice on examination technique, as well as specific questions carefully structured to test your ability and to help you to appreciate the standard required. To gain full benefit from what is provided here, you will need the help of a more senior anaesthetist to advise you on the quality of your written answers and the co-operation of a colleague who is also studying for the exam or who has recently taken it, to enable the material provided in relation to the Clinical Oral, to be used to create the situation of a 'Mock Viva'.

The answer sections have all been gathered at the end of the book, to try to discourage any tendency to read the answers before the questions!

THE PART 1 FFARCS EXAMINATION

There are four sections:

1. 60 Multiple True/False questions — 2 hours
2. Seven compulsory essays — 3 hours
3. Clinical Oral - using guided questions — 30 minutes
4. Oral - including physics of equipment — 30 minutes

STANDARD REQUIRED
The following guidance is given: "The Faculty is looking for a level of performance which will distinguish a safe practitioner, able to handle any emergency without unnecessary further deterioration for a limited time until more experienced or skilled help can be obtained, and one who understands the extent of his abilities and the circumstances in which assistance needs to be sought.

Thus, as well as giving correct answers, the successful candidate will give them with some confidence and promptness and will demonstrate good judgement by dealing with real problems rather than some perceived theoretical problems. The successful candidate, in short, is someone the examiner would be prepared to see promoted to a registrar post in a District General Hospital."

The key words are 'safe practitioner' and 'good judgement' and the inference to be drawn is that when presented with questions, especially in the Orals, that relate to clinical situations one should always adopt a sensible and cautious approach, based upon the principles described in the standard anaesthetic textbooks.

SYLLABUS
Unlike the other parts of the FFA examination, considerable information is given about the syllabus for the Part 1.

"This examination will cover those aspects of anaesthetic practice relevant to the introductory first year of training in anaesthesia, including anaesthetic aspects of the management of acute medical and surgical emergencies.

The relevant subjects are:
Anaesthesia for general surgery, orthopaedics and trauma, principles of obstetric anaesthesia and analgesia, anaesthesia for children (but not neonates), gynaecology and urology, ophthalmology, otorhinolaryngology, dentistry; commonly used regional anaesthetic techniques, immediate care and resuscitation, recovery room practice, physical principles related to the working of anaesthetic equipment and lung ventilators. The candidate is not expected to have detailed knowledge of anaesthesia for

neonatal, thoracic and neuro-surgery, or of intensive therapy or pain relief (other than in the early postoperative period). Examination in physiology and pharmacology at an advanced level takes place in the Part 2 (Basic Science) and in the Part 3 (Final) examinations, but the Part 1 examination includes:

Physiology
Applied aspects of physiology relevant to basic anaesthetic practice, and to medicine and surgery related to anaesthesia.

Pharmacology
The applied pharmacology of drugs relevant to basic anaesthetic practice with an understanding of chemical properties, relevant formulation, side effects, drug interactions and the elements of pharmacokinetics.

Physics
Elementary physics related to techniques and apparatus. Monitoring for routine anaesthesia.

Anatomy
Anatomy related to the practice of general anaesthesia and commonly used regional anaesthetic techniques.

Medicine and Surgery
Aspects of medicine and surgery relevant to anaesthesia for elective and emergency surgery (but with the exclusion of specialist topics already mentioned). Preoperative assessment, preparation and medication, immediate postoperative care, and the recognition and treatment of postoperative complications related to anaesthesia, resuscitation and immediate care."

It may well be that many candidates will not have had direct involvement with some of the types of surgery that are specified and it is important to identify any deficiencies in one's experience and to be sure that these topics are covered in preparing for the exam. Obstetrics and anaesthesia for children are not usually regarded as being within the competence of a first year SHO, but they are included in the syllabus and to be "someone the examiner would be prepared to see promoted to a registrar post in a District General Hospital", it is necessary to be able to show an awareness of the potential problems in these areas as well as a knowledge of how they should be managed. The inclusion of commonly used regional anaesthetic techniques in the syllabus is often not appreciated by candidates who have failed to prepare for the questions that are asked.

MARKING SYSTEM

Close marking systems are used in most medical examinations, but for the Part 1 the grading method is particularly tight.

    2+   Good pass
    2   Pass
    1+   Marginal fail
    1   Bad fail
    0   Veto

The effect of such close marking is that a 1 or even a 1+ in any part can be very difficult to recover from. To pass, candidates should try to achieve a good average standard in all the parts of the examination.

THE MULTIPLE CHOICE QUESTION PAPER

The use of MCQ papers is now so widespread in medical examinations that anyone sitting the Part 1 FFA will without doubt have met them before, but it is important to remember their advantages and disadvantages. Unlike essays and orals which tend to be subjective, MCQ's enable an objective test of factual knowledge to be made over a wide area of the syllabus. They can however be criticised for being a superficial test, for they do not assess the ability to weigh up the relative importance of information as may be required in clinical situations.

In some subjects, pharmacology for instance, it is not difficult to structure unambiguous MCQ's, whereas in clinical anaesthesia where things are less clear cut and exceptions abound, the setting of questions is less easy. Take this into account, trust the examiner and do not look for ambiguities and difficulties that do not exist. Some candidates read the questions as if they are legal experts and quote obscure references to justify their answer. Forget it, take the questions at face value do not look for difficulties that are not there.

QUESTION STRUCTURE
Each question is of the multiple true or false format and consists of a stem and five branches, each of which in conjunction with the stem is either a true or a false statement. Candidates have to state for each response whether it is true or false. They may choose not to answer.

Take care not to let your answer to one branch influence your answers to the other branches. Re-read the stem each time in conjunction with the individual branch as a complete statement. If this is not done it is easy to make errors, especially in situations where negatives are used in either the stem or branch, or worst of all if there are negatives in both.

MARKING
"Candidates receive +1 mark for each correctly answered response, −1 for each response incorrectly answered and 0 if no attempt is made to answer." Therefore the maximum for each question if all 5 are right is +5, and if all incorrect the minimum is −5.

A raw score is then worked out from the total number of the correct true or false answers, less the total number of incorrect true or false answers, this raw score could be negative. The percentage score on which assessment is based, is the raw score multiplied by 100 and divided by the maximum possible score, which in this exam is 300. It is known that 'discriminator questions' are used, these are questions that have been set previously and the candidates' performance in these can be compared with their use on previous occasions. On the basis of this the pass mark for the whole exam can be adjusted to compensate for any variation in the overall ease or difficulty of the remaining questions.

PASS MARK
The MCQ paper acts as a screen, and about 10-15% of candidates are excluded from the Orals because of their poor performance in the MCQ, exceptionally if their performance is really dreadful, they "may be referred for one year" before they can attempt the exam again. It is probable that the pass mark generally lies around 55-60% and making allowance for the fact that a variable proportion of one's answers will be wrong, it seems unlikely that a candidate will pass if less than 200 answers are filled in on the computer card. For those not excluded from the rest of the exam on their MCQ performance alone, there is always the opportunity of improving a marginal MCQ mark with a good performance in the rest of the examination.

GUESSING
Wild guesses should be randomly correct or incorrect and should lead to a score of zero, so guessing is unlikely to improve your score. There is however what can be called the informed guess or hunch, it is generally agreed that if you are only moderately sure of an answer it usually better to follow your hunch rather than to leave the question unanswered.

WORDING OF QUESTIONS
It cannot be said too often that it is vital to read each question carefully, re-reading the stem with each branch. The wording of the questions has been done with considerable care and each word is there for a reason. There are however certain 'weasel words' that often cause problems and should be treated with care. 'Always' and 'never' can rarely be used in relation to questions about clinical problems and therefore words such as 'commonly', 'rarely', 'may' and suchlike abound in MCQ papers. Try not to let yourself become obsessed by them. Trust those who set the paper and do not look for tricks. If a question seems ambiguous and you are genuinely confused by the wording, an examiner is usually present at the examination and you should ask him for clarification.

Good false answers are particularly difficult to devise, often they are based on the opposite of the right answer, look carefully to be sure that prefixes such as hyper- and hypo- are really correct. The genuine red herring can be difficult to check as one often feels that if you read widely enough you will find a reference showing it to be correct, but at the level of the Part 1 FFA if it is not in the standard textbooks the answer can be taken as wrong.

The Multiple Choice Question Paper

FILLING IN ANSWERS
"At each examination candidates receive a question book detailing the questions and a printed lector sheet on which they mark their answers. Candidates are not allowed to retain the question book. They are advised, in the examination instructions, to enter their answers in the question book first and then to transpose them to the lector sheet."

The so-called lector sheet or computer card should be marked exactly according to the instructions and with great care. They are marked by being passed through an automatic document reader and untidiness can lead to the machine misreading the answer.

PLAN OF CAMPAIGN
Although everyone will have their own way of organising their time during the paper, we give here a suggested 'plan of campaign'. Whether or not you choose to use it, we believe that it is a good idea to consider it carefully so that you have thought about your own approach before you enter the examination hall.

1. Fill in your name, number or other details that are required on the computer card.

2. Go through the paper steadily doing the following:

    a) mark on *the question paper* the answers to those questions of which you are sure of the answer, by putting for instance a T for true and F for false against each branch.
    b) put a line through any question if you feel that you have no clue about the subject or the correct answers.
    c) put a question mark by the stem of the remaining questions, these are those that you believe you could answer given time to think about them.

3. Check the time and work out how much is left leaving aside at least half an hour to fill in the computer card, then count up the number of questions you have put a question mark by and work out how much time you can therefore spend on each question.

4. Go through the paper again trying to work out the answers to the marked questions but not spending more than the calculated proportion of time on any one.

5. Check the time, there should still be plenty left. Mark the computer card exactly as instructed, double checking to ensure that you are doing so correctly. Mistakes can be made by getting out of phase

between the number of the question in the paper and on the computer card, it is therefore sensible to mark say five questions at a time and then check them to ensure that both the marking and their numbers are correct. *It is vital that the marking on to the computer card is done correctly.*

6. Finally, go back to any question that you felt you might have puzzled out with more time, but resist the temptation to change the answers to other questions unless you are absolutely sure that the original answer was wrong. Mark these on the computer card as you go.

Check once more that your name and number are on the computer card before handing it in. With an MCQ exam, if you feel you have done all the questions you can, it is best to leave the examination hall.

DISTRIBUTION OF QUESTIONS
We are told that "both the MCQ and the essays will cover a full range of relevant basic sciences set in the context of clinical experience appropriate to one year's practical training." Thus there will be questions which have a physiological, anatomical, medical, pharmacological or therapeutic bias in both written parts of the examination. Beyond this there is no further guidance but the balance of questions in the MCQ paper is probably about:

  20 anaesthetics
  12 pharmacology
   4 physics and clinical measurement
   2 anatomy
  12 physiology
  10 medicine and surgery

This has been used as the basis of the test MCQ papers in this book.

HOW TO USE THE MCQ PAPERS IN THIS BOOK
We would suggest that you work through each of these sets of 60 multiple choice questions as if it were a real examination. To do this you should spend no more than 90 minutes on each, this will ensure that sufficient time is allowed in the real examination to fill in the answers on the computer cards. Try to reproduce examination conditions as closely as possible by being sure you will not be disturbed and resisting any temptation to obtain help from books.

As you work through each question be sure and mark your answer against the space by the A... B... C... D... E... at the bottom, using 'T' for True and 'F' for False. When you have completed the paper you can then mark it by using the answers at the back of the book. If you wish you can give yourself

The Multiple Choice Question Paper

+1 for each correct answer and −1 for each incorrect answer and thus work out your raw score and corrected percentage score in the way described in the previous section.

Rather than worrying too much about your score, the explanations and references to standard text books should be used to identify and remedy any gaps in your knowledge.

MCQ : PRACTICE EXAM 1

60 Questions: Time allowed 2 hours
Indicate your answers by writing T for True and F for False
in the spaces provided.

1   At equivalent MAC, comparing halothane with enflurane

   A   enflurane causes more respiratory depression than halothane
   B   enflurane causes more cardiac arrhythmias than halothane
   C   enflurane causes a greater fall in cardiac output than halothane
   D   similar amounts of inorganic fluoride are produced in the metabolism of both agents
   E   enflurane has a higher boiling point than halothane

   Your answers: A.......B.......C.......D.......E.......

2   The following are true of intravenous regional anaesthesia:

   A   it was first described by Carl August Bier in 1908 using lignocaine
   B   in the arm a cannula for the injection of local anaesthetic may safely be placed in the antecubital fossa
   C   the tourniquet should be inflated to 30 mmHg above systolic pressure
   D   bupivacaine 0.125% is a suitable agent to use
   E   it should not be used in patients with sickle cell trait

   Your answers: A.......B.......C.......D.......E.......

3   Soda lime

   A   is mainly calcium carbonate
   B   can be used to scavenge nitrous oxide
   C   needs water to absorb carbon dioxide
   D   in a properly packed cannister half the volume should be space between the granules
   E   gets hot in use

   Your answers: A.......B.......C.......D.......E.......

4   In anaesthesia for the evacuation of retained products of conception, the following drugs at concentrations normally used for anaesthesia, can cause a reduction of uterine tone:

   A   halothane
   B   enflurane
   C   thiopentone and nitrous oxide
   D   cyclopropane
   E   ketamine

   Your answers: A.......B.......C.......D.......E.......

MCQ Exam 1

5 Following intravenous thiopentone, the following may occur:

A severe hypotension
B respiratory depression
C liver toxicity
D increased intracranial pressure
E epileptic convulsions

Your answers: A.......B.......C.......D.......E.......

6 A new anaesthetic agent has a saturated vapour pressure at 20°C of 152 mmHg. If there is a total fresh gas flow of 4 l/min of which 80 ml/min is diverted through the vaporiser, the inspired concentration will be approximately

A 1.6%
B 0.8%
C 2%
D 0.5%
E 5%

Your answers: A.......B.......C.......D.......E.......

7 In a hypertensive patient for anaesthesia on treatment with clonidine

A calcium supplements need to be given
B clonidine should be withdrawn 6 hours prior to anaesthesia
C anaemia may be present as a result of bone marrow depression
D halothane is contraindicated
E if the blood pressure falls intra-operatively a noradrenaline infusion is required

Your answers: A.......B.......C.......D.......E.......

8 The following anaesthetic induction agents commonly cause thrombosis on intravenous injection:

A thiopentone
B etomidate
C methohexitone
D diazepam in propylene glycol
E diazemuls

Your answers: A.......B.......C.......D.......E.......

MCQ Exam 1

9 **Recognised complications of supraclavicular brachial plexus block include**

A intravascular administration of local anaesthetic
B pneumothorax
C vagal block
D phrenic nerve block
E Horner's syndrome

Your answers: A.......B.......C.......D.......E.......

10 **Convulsions occurring intra-operatively or in the early postoperative period may be due to**

A ether
B suxamethonium
C halothane
D bupivacaine
E hypoxia

Your answers: A.......B.......C.......D.......E.......

11 **The Magill circuit**

A is an example of a Mapleson A circuit
B is functionally similar to the Lack circuit
C is suitable for children over 25 kg
D is suitable for IPPV
E rebreathing and hypercarbia will occur if the fresh gas flow is less than the minute volume

Your answers: A.......B.......C.......D.......E.......

12 **Useful tests of clinically adequate return of muscle power after neuromuscular block include**

A head lift sustained for 5 seconds
B measurement of tidal volume
C measurement of minute volume
D measurement of end tidal CO_2
E assessing the response to airway obstruction

Your answers: A.......B.......C.......D.......E.......

MCQ Exam 1

13 Which of the following pathology results should lead to postponement of a routine operation and further investigation:

   A haemoglobin 10.8 g/dl
   B glycosuria
   C serum potassium 5.0 mmol/l
   D porphyrinuria
   E bilirubin 15 µmol/l

   Your answers: A.......B.......C.......D.......E.......

14 Arrhythmias at induction of anaesthesia may be

   A the result of the use of topical lignocaine in the larynx
   B due to the volatile anaesthetic agent
   C the result of sympatho-autonomic reflexes
   D more common in hypertensive patients
   E reduced by preoperative β-blockers

   Your answers: A.......B.......C.......D.......E.......

15 A tourniquet to achieve a bloodless field for surgery of the lower limb

   A should not be inflated for more than one hour
   B should be inflated to 50 mmHg above the systolic blood pressure
   C is associated with an increased risk of postoperative deep vein thrombosis
   D should not be used under spinal anaesthesia
   E is contraindicated in the presence of HbS

   Your answers: A.......B.......C.......D.......E.......

16 In an elderly patient with a fractured hip who is in poor health

   A it is reasonable to delay the operation for 7-10 days
   B the most common cause of death is pulmonary embolism
   C the choice of anaesthetic technique has no bearing on post-operative mortality in the first two weeks
   D clinically significant arterial hypoxaemia follows any anaesthetic technique
   E spinal block to T10 is adequate

   Your answers: A.......B.......C.......D.......E.......

MCQ Exam 1

17 The following may be useful in the treatment of malignant hyperpyrexia:

    A   calcium EDTA
    B   sodium EDTA
    C   dantrolene sodium
    D   mannitol
    E   magnesium sulphate

Your answers: A.......B.......C.......D.......E.......

18 The following are true of minimum alveolar concentration, MAC:

    A   enflurane is greater than isoflurane
    B   methoxyflurane is greater than halothane
    C   cyclopropane is greater than isoflurane
    D   nitrous oxide is greater than one atmosphere
    E   it correlates with the blood/gas partition coefficient

Your answers: A.......B.......C.......D.......E.......

19 The following are explosive at concentrations usually used for general anaesthesia:

    A   cyclopropane
    B   halothane
    C   ether
    D   enflurane
    E   methoxyflurane

Your answers: A.......B.......C.......D.......E.......

20 A fit 50 year old man develops a slow nodal rhythm during halothane anaesthesia

    A   this is dangerous and requires treatment
    B   this is often induced by a fall in blood pressure
    C   it may be due to hypoxia
    D   it is often associated with light anaesthesia
    E   this usually responds to intravenous atropine

Your answers: A.......B.......C.......D.......E.......

MCQ Exam 1

21 Digoxin is indicated in

    A   atrial flutter
    B   2:1 block
    C   ventricular tachycardia
    D   nodal tachycardia
    E   Stokes-Adams attacks

Your answers: A.......B.......C.......D.......E.......

22 Dopamine infused at a dosage of 10μg/kg/minute would produce

    A   increased urinary output
    B   increased sodium excretion
    C   increased cardiac output
    D   multiple ventricular extrasystoles
    E   an unchanged peripheral resistance

Your answers: A.......B.......C.......D.......E.......

23 Ketamine

    A   raises intracranial pressure
    B   causes muscle relaxation
    C   relaxes the uterus
    D   is excreted in the urine
    E   premedication with atropine is essential when it is used

Your answers: A.......B.......C.......D.......E.......

24 The blood glucose may be lowered by

    A   isoprenaline
    B   growth hormone
    C   metformin
    D   glucagon
    E   glibenclamide

Your answers: A.......B.......C.......D.......E.......

MCQ Exam 1

25 Sodium dantrolene

A is a neuromuscular blocker
B may cause dangerous rises in the serum calcium
C can be used preoperatively to reduce suxamethonium pains
D is useful in the treatment of malignant hyperpyrexia
E is a skeletal muscle relaxant

Your answers: A.......B.......C.......D.......E.......

26 Isoflurane

A has the same molecular weight as enflurane
B if put in a calibrated halothane vaporiser (e.g. Fluotec), it will deliver dangerously high concentrations of isoflurane
C reduces the blood pressure mainly by depressing cardiac output
D has a MAC of 1.68%
E causes minimal changes in cerebral blood flow at light levels of anaesthesia (up to 1 MAC)

Your answers: A.......B.......C.......D.......E.......

27 Naloxone can be used to reverse respiratory depression caused by

A thiopentone
B nalbuphine
C pentazocine
D phenobarbitone
E oxazepam

Your answers: A.......B.......C.......D.......E.......

28 The following are true of thiopentone:

A the pH of a 2.5% solution is 6.8
B less than 15% of an administered dose is metabolised each hour
C it is the sulphur analogue of pentobarbitone
D it is more than 50% protein bound
E it exists in the plasma in both ionised and non-ionised forms

Your answers: A.......B.......C.......D.......E.......

MCQ Exam 1

29 In comparison with atropine, hyoscine

    A is more anti-emetic
    B induces more tachycardia
    C is more sedative
    D is a more effective anti-sialogogue
    E has a greater anti-Parkinsonian action

Your answers: A.......B.......C.......D.......E.......

30 Depolarising muscle blockade with suxamethonium is characterised by

    A potentiation by neostigmine
    B antagonism with d-tubocurarine
    C fade
    D post-tetanic facilitation
    E antagonism by lowering body temperature

Your answers: A.......B.......C.......D.......E.......

31 The following can cause dependence with prolonged administration:

    A morphine
    B pentazocine
    C phenylbutazone
    D quinalbarbitone
    E pethidine

Your answers: A.......B.......C.......D.......E.......

32 Bupivacaine

    A produces depolarisation in the neural membrane of peripheral nerves
    B is detoxified in the liver
    C is an ester
    D can cause methaemoglobinaemia
    E 30 ml of 0.5% solution is the recommended maximum dose in a fit 75 kg man

Your answers: A.......B.......C.......D.......E.......

MCQ Exam 1

33 The following may lead to over-estimation of the blood pressure:

  A   too wide a cuff
  B   too fat an arm and a standard cuff
  C   letting the cuff down too slowly
  D   having the sphygmomanometer above the patient
  E   severe atherosclerosis

  Your answers: A.......B.......C.......D.......E.......

34 The critical pressure is

  A   the maximum pressure to which a cylinder can be filled
  B   the pressure above which a liquid cannot evaporate
  C   the pressure at which a vapour is in equilibrium with its liquid
  D   120 bar
  E   the pressure at which a gas ignites

  Your answers: A.......B.......C.......D.......E.......

35 For laminar flow in a tube, the flow rate is directly proportional to

  A   its length
  B   the fourth power of its radius
  C   the density of the gas or liquid flowing through it
  D   the pressure drop across it
  E   the viscosity of the gas or liquid flowing through it

  Your answers: A.......B.......C.......D.......E.......

36 Helium has the following advantages over nitrogen for divers at depth:

  A   it diffuses more rapidly into the body tissues
  B   it is denser
  C   it has a lower viscosity
  D   it has less narcotic effect
  E   it is a good insulator

  Your answers: A.......B.......C.......D.......E.......

17

MCQ Exam 1

37 The basilic vein

- A arises on the palmar aspect of the hand
- B passes up the radial side of the forearm
- C goes through the clavipectoral fascia between the deltoid and pectoralis major muscles
- D runs with the radial nerve
- E becomes the axillary vein

Your answers: A.......B.......C.......D.......E.......

38 In relation to the first rib

- A scalenus medius inserts into the scalene tubercle
- B the lower trunk of the brachial plexus lies on the upper surface
- C the subclavian artery lies in front of the scalene tubercle
- D the stellate ganglion lies anterior to its head
- E the subclavian vein lies behind the scalene tubercle

Your answers: A.......B.......C.......D.......E.......

39 A Valsalva manoeuvre

- A is a forced expiration against a closed glottis or other airway obstruction
- B is initially associated with increased systolic arterial pressure
- C is associated with a decreased total peripheral resistance
- D is normally associated with a tachycardia
- E is normally followed by a bradycardia

Your answers: A.......B.......C.......D.......E.......

40 Albumin

- A has a molecular weight of approximately 65,000
- B is increased in chronic liver disease
- C is increased in malabsorption syndrome
- D makes a significant contribution to plasma oncotic pressure
- E has a normal value of 34-45 g/l

Your answers: A.......B.......C.......D.......E.......

MCQ Exam 1

41 The minute volume is

    A   reduced during sleep
    B   reduced by a rise in body temperature
    C   reduced by an increase in body acidity
    D   increased by hypothermia
    E   increased by arrival at a height of 5,000 metres

Your answers: A.......B.......C.......D.......E.......

42 The haemoglobin oxygen dissociation curve is moved to the right by

    A   acidosis
    B   raised body temperature
    C   passage through the pulmonary capillaries
    D   ageing
    E   anaemia

Your answers: A.......B.......C.......D.......E.......

43 The knee jerk

    A   arises from the spinal cord at T12
    B   is controlled by higher centres
    C   results from stimulation of the intrafusal fibres
    D   results from stimulation of the Golgi tendon organ
    E   is a monosynaptic reflex

Your answers: A.......B.......C.......D.......E.......

44 Carbon dioxide is transported in the blood

    A   in the red cells
    B   as phosphate esters
    C   in simple solution
    D   combined with plasma protein
    E   as carbamino compound with haemoglobin

Your answers: A.......B.......C.......D.......E.......

MCQ Exam 1

45 Acclimatisation to the hypoxia of high altitude results in

  A a decreased affinity of haemoglobin for oxygen
  B a reduced arterial CO_2 level
  C an increase in oxygen carrying capacity
  D an increase in respiratory minute volume
  E an increase in cardiac output

  Your answers: A.......B.......C.......D.......E.......

46 In the normal heart

  A the resting membrane potential is -80 mV
  B the PR interval is greater than 0.2 sec
  C the PR interval represents the period between sinoatrial depolarisation and atrial contraction
  D the T wave represents ventricular repolarisation
  E the S wave occurs at the start of diastole

  Your answers: A.......B.......C.......D.......E.......

47 In a normally hydrated healthy man
  A the GFR is approximately 125 ml/min
  B urinary pH is an accurate reflection of blood pH
  C the urinary sodium is in the range 50-200 mmol/24 hours
  D the urinary osmolality is in the range 100-1500 mosmol/kg
  E creatinine clearance is a reliable indication of GFR

  Your answers: A.......B.......C.......D.......E.......

48 In a recording of the central venous pressure

  A the 'a' wave is caused by atrial systole
  B the 'c' wave is caused by bulging of the tricuspid valve during isometric ventricular contraction
  C the 'v' wave is due to atrial filling with the tricuspid valve closed
  D the pressure is increased during inspiration
  E the pressure is always raised if left atrial pressure is increased

  Your answers: A.......B.......C.......D.......E.......

MCQ Exam 1

49 **The functional residual capacity (FRC)**

A falls with age
B falls under anaesthesia with spontaneous respiration
C rises under anaesthesia with IPPV
D when it is reduced, the difference between the alveolar and arterial oxygen tension is reduced
E if it falls below closing capacity, atelectasis will ensue

Your answers: A.......B.......C.......D.......E.......

50 **The following are true in regard of arterial blood gases:**

A the normal hydrogen ion concentration is 100 nmol/l
B the normal standard bicarbonate is 32 mmol/l
C a PO_2 of 10 kPa (75 mmHg) is normal for an 80 year old man
D the PCO_2 is raised in hypothermia
E the base deficit is the number of mmol of bicarbonate per litre of blood, required to correct the pH to 7.4 at a PCO_2 of 5.3 kPa (40 mmHg) and 37°C

Your answers: A.......B.......C.......D.......E.......

51 **Raynaud's phenomenon**

A can occur in the toes as well as the fingers
B is associated with cryoglobulinaemia
C invariably responds to vasodilators
D may lead to irreversible ischaemic changes
E invariably responds to sympathectomy

Your answers: A.......B.......C.......D.......E.......

52 **Chronic deficiency of hormones of the adrenal cortex is associated with**

A low serum sodium
B the appearance of striae on the abdomen
C low blood pressure
D loss of skin pigmentation
E low serum potassium

Your answers: A.......B.......C.......D.......E.......

MCQ Exam 1

53 Chronic bronchitis is characterised by

    A   air trapping in the alveolae
    B   increased mucus secretion
    C   a reduced residual volume
    D   a normal ratio between forced expiratory volume (FEV_1) and forced vital capacity (FVC)
    E   maximum life expectancy of 10 years

Your answers: A.......B.......C......D.......E.......

54 Angina pectoris is a recognised feature of

    A   aortic stenosis
    B   anaemia
    C   polyarteritis
    D   myxoedema
    E   paroxysmal ventricular tachycardia

Your answers: A.......B.......C......D.......E.......

55 Glycine 1.5% used for irrigation during trans-urethral prostatectomy (TURP) can cause

    A   hyponatraemia
    B   hypercalcaemia
    C   haemolysis
    D   hyperkalaemia
    E   haemodilution

Your answers: A.......B.......C......D.......E.......

56 On the ECG, P-waves are always seen in

    A   atrial flutter
    B   ventricular tachycardia
    C   nodal rhythm
    D   complete heart block
    E   supraventricular tachycardia

Your answers: A.......B.......C......D.......E.......

MCQ Exam 1

57 Plasma values of potassium 6.5 mmol and sodium 125 mmol may be seen in

   A   oliguric renal failure
   B   hypopituitarism
   C   adreno-cortical insufficiency
   D   Cushing's syndrome
   E   primary hyperaldosteronism (Conn's syndrome)

   Your answers: A.......B.......C.......D.......E.......

58 The presence of gallstones is associated with

   A   carcinoma of the gall bladder
   B   intolerance to alcohol
   C   cholangitis
   D   pancreatitis
   E   intestinal obstruction

   Your answers: A.......B.......C.......D.......E.......

59 In comparison with patients suffering mainly from emphysema (pink puffers), those whose disease is primarily due to chronic bronchitis (blue bloaters) have a

   A   lower arterial PCO_2
   B   higher standard bicarbonate
   C   lower haematocrit
   D   lower arterial PO_2
   E   lower diffusing capacity for carbon monoxide (transfer factor)

   Your answers: A.......B.......C.......D.......E.......

60 In patients with sickle cell trait (heterozygotes)

   A   a Sickledex test will allow differentiation from homozygotes
   B   moderate anaemia is usually present
   C   episodic haematuria may be seen
   D   splenomegaly is a characteristic finding
   E   exchange transfusion may be necessary for major thoracic surgery

   Your answers: A.......B.......C.......D.......E.......

END OF PRACTICE EXAM 1

Go over your answers until your time is up.
Answers and explanations are on page 87.

MCQ PRACTICE EXAM 2

60 Questions: Time allowed 2 hours
Indicate your answers by writing T for True and F for False
in the spaces provided.

1 At concentrations normally used for clinical anaesthesia, halothane

   A is inflammable
   B raises the intracranial pressure
   C cannot be used in a closed circuit with soda lime
   D sensitises the heart to the effect of catecholamines
   E relaxes the uterus

   Your answers: A....... B....... C....... D....... E.......

2 Intubation of the right main bronchus with unchanged ventilation may in the first 5 minutes, lead to

   A hypotension
   B hypercapnia
   C an increased requirement for an insoluble anaesthetic agent
   D collapse of the right upper lobe
   E hypoxaemia

   Your answers: A....... B....... C....... D....... E.......

3 In malignant hyperpyrexia

   A the creatine phosphokinase (CPK) is raised
   B there may be rigidity following suxamethonium administration
   C rigidity can be relieved by 5 mg of d-tubocurarine
   D muscle tissue is histologically abnormal
   E the onset may be during recovery

   Your answers: A....... B....... C....... D....... E.......

4 Depolarising block may be produced by

   A suxamethonium
   B neostigmine
   C atracurium
   D gallamine
   E edrophonium

   Your answers: A....... B....... C....... D....... E.......

MCQ Exam 2

5 The following are halogenated ethers:

    A   methoxyflurane
    B   cyclopropane
    C   enflurane
    D   halothane
    E   isoflurane

Your answers: A.......B.......C.......D.......E.......

6 At normal anaesthetic concentrations trichlorethylene

    A   is highly volatile
    B   is a vasodilator
    C   is very irritant to the respiratory tract
    D   can cause tachypnoea
    E   should not be used with soda lime

Your answers: A.......B.......C.......D.......E.......

7 A patient 4 hours postoperatively shows the following:- BP 170/100, pulse 100, warm periphery, arterial blood gases on air PCO_2 9.0, PO_2 9.0 and bicarbonate 28 mmol, this may be due to

    A   segmental pulmonary collapse
    B   septicaemia
    C   overtransfusion
    D   underventilation
    E   metabolic acidosis

Your answers: A.......B.......C.......D.......E.......

8 In lignocaine overdosage, the following may occur:

    A   unconsciousness
    B   hypotension
    C   involuntary movements
    D   bronchospasm
    E   hypothermia

Your answers: A.......B.......C.......D.......E.......

MCQ Exam 2

9 **Warming blood to 37°C for massive blood transfusion**

    A   reduces the incidence of infection
    B   increases the CO_2 tension
    C   reduces the O_2 tension
    D   shifts the oxygen dissociation curve to the right
    E   reduces the incidence of arrhythmias

Your answers: A.......B.......C.......D.......E.......

10 **The following commonly cause pain on intravenous injection into small veins:**

    A   etomidate
    B   methohexitone
    C   neostigmine
    D   suxamethonium
    E   d-tubocurarine

Your answers: A.......B.......C.......D.......E.......

11 **Severely obese patients may be**

    A   hypoxaemic
    B   difficult to intubate
    C   unusually sensitive to non-depolarising muscle relaxants
    D   unusually sensitive to thiopentone
    E   hypercarbic

Your answers: A.......B.......C.......D.......E.......

12 **When testing a modern Boyles machine, e.g. the Boyle International, prior to use**

    A   the pipelines should remain connected at all times
    B   disconnection of nitrous oxide supply prevents the functioning of the oxygen failure alarm
    C   vaporisers should be turned on when testing for leaks
    D   occluding the anaesthetic gas outlet should lead to the pressure blow off valve opening
    E   a Tritec vaporiser cannot be turned on with the closed circuit

Your answers: A.......B.......C.......D.......E.......

MCQ Exam 2

13 Recognised complications of dextran infusions are

   A antigenic reactions
   B problems with the cross-matching of blood
   C an increase in venous thrombosis
   D renal failure
   E an increase in rouleaux formation of the red cells

   Your answers: A.......B.......C.......D.......E.......

14 The level of serum potassium may be

   A increased by suxamethonium
   B increased by thiopentone
   C increased in metabolic alkalosis
   D affected by extensive burns
   E reduced by d-tubocurarine

   Your answers: A.......B.......C.......D.......E.......

15 Fat embolism may produce

   A fat in the sputum
   B fat in the urine
   C petechial haemorrhages
   D pyrexia
   E respiratory distress

   Your answers: A.......B.......C.......D.......E.......

16 Non-depolarising muscle relaxants

   A produce post-tetanic facilitation
   B all have their action prolonged by alkalosis
   C produce fasciculation
   D can exhibit dual block
   E have a prolonged action in severe hypothermia

   Your answers: A.......B.......C.......D.......E.......

MCQ Exam 2

17 With medical oxygen

A the critical temperature is 36.5°C
B manufacture is by the fractional distillation of air
C explosions can occur if, under pressure, it comes into contact with oil or grease
D convulsions can be caused if it is given under hyperbaric conditions
E bone marrow depression can occur with prolonged administration

Your answers: A........B........C........D........E........

18 In Guedel's classification of the depth of anaesthesia

A there are four stages
B there are 4 planes in stage 3
C the classification was based on open ether and spontaneous respiration
D in stage 2 respiration is regular
E the pupils are small in stage 2

Your answers: A........B........C........D........E........

19 In nitrous oxide cylinders for medical use

A the cylinder is initially full of liquid
B nitrous oxide is produced by heating ammonium nitrate
C contaminants may be tested for with moistened starch-iodide paper
D in continuous use the gauge pressure will only fall when the cylinder is nearly empty
E contamination with nitric oxide may occur

Your answers: A........B........C........D........E........

20 The following are true in relation to caudal block:

A it is an extradural injection through the sacrococcygeal membrane
B the dura extends down to the lower border of L5
C it causes some parasympathetic blockade
D bupivacaine 0.25%, 0.5 ml/kg is a suitable dose for children having circumcision under general anaesthesia
E the average capacity of the sacral canal is 24 ml in adult males

Your answers: A........B........C........D........E........

MCQ Exam 2

21 The following reduce airways resistance in asthmatics:

    A aminophylline
    B propranolol
    C salbutamol
    D isoprenaline
    E aldosterone

Your answers: A.......B.......C.......D.......E.......

22 The following act on peripheral α-adrenergic receptors:

    A clonidine
    B phenoxybenzamine
    C trimetaphan
    D droperidol
    E phentolamine

Your answers: A.......B.......C.......D.......E.......

23 Pancuronium

    A is less likely than d-tubocurarine to cause a fall in blood pressure
    B causes a rise in heart rate
    C is potentiated by streptomycin
    D does not cross the placenta in clinically significant concentration
    E is excreted only through the kidneys

Your answers: A.......B.......C.......D.......E.......

24 Morphine

    A may cause histamine release
    B decreases catecholamine levels
    C causes miosis
    D causes vomiting by direct stimulation of vomiting centre
    E arterial PCO_2 is markedly raised with normal therapeutic dosage

Your answers: A.......B.......C.......D.......E.......

MCQ Exam 2

25 Chlorpromazine

- A   is a weak antihistamine
- B   is an α-blocker
- C   can cause Parkinsonism
- D   is an anti-emetic
- E   has an atropine-like action

Your answers: A.......B.......C.......D.......E.......

26 The MAC value of an inhalational anaesthetic agent will be influenced by

- A   the age of the patient
- B   the administration of morphine with it
- C   changes in the arterial PCO_2 from 3.5 to 6.5 kPa (26 to 49 mmHg)
- D   its blood/gas partition coefficient
- E   the use of nitrous oxide with it

Your answers: A.......B.......C.......D.......E.......

27 Halothane decreases the blood pressure as a result of

- A   direct myocardial depression
- B   a fall in total peripheral resistance
- C   a central action on the vasomotor centre
- D   ganglion blockade
- E   increased aldosterone secretion

Your answers: A.......B.......C.......D.......E.......

28 The following are anticonvulsant:

- A   diazepam
- B   chlormethiazole
- C   oxazepam
- D   chlorpropamide
- E   thiopentone

Your answers: A.......B.......C.......D.......E.......

MCQ Exam 2

29 **Propranolol is contraindicated in**

    A   bronchial asthma
    B   the presence of a low serum potassium
    C   paroxysmal nocturnal dyspnoea
    D   patients already on digoxin
    E   atrial fibrillation

Your answers: A.......B.......C.......D.......E.......

30 **Significant vasoconstriction occurs with**

    A   cocaine
    B   amethocaine
    C   prilocaine
    D   lignocaine
    E   bupivacaine

Your answers: A.......B.......C.......D.......E.......

31 **Methohexitone**

    A   is not a barbiturate
    B   is less potent than thiopentone
    C   is contraindicated in acute intermittent porphyria
    D   is excreted unchanged in the urine
    E   can cause excitatory movements

Your answers: A.......B.......C.......D.......E.......

32 **Chlorpropamide**

    A   has a half life of 12 hours
    B   is mainly metabolised in the liver
    C   causes alcohol intolerance in about 30% of patients
    D   acts by stimulating insulin production
    E   results in unwanted effects twice as commonly as tolbutamide

Your answers: A.......B.......C.......D.......E.......

MCQ Exam 2

33 The following are true for gases in cylinders:

- A oxygen is stored at 120 lbf/sq in
- B nitrous oxide is stored at 51 lbf/sq in
- C nitrous oxide should contain 1% water vapour
- D nitrous oxide should not be stored below -8°C.
- E size E cylinders of oxygen and nitrous oxide are generally used on a Boyles machine

Your answers: A.......B.......C.......D.......E.......

34 The accuracy of a rotameter may be affected by

- A dirt on the bobbin
- B static electricity
- C passing the wrong gas through it
- D back pressure from a Manley ventilator
- E using it at high altitude

Your answers: A.......B.......C.......D.......E.......

35 The critical temperature is

- A the temperature at which a gas becomes liquid if the pressure is raised
- B the temperature above which a gas cannot be liquefied by increasing pressure alone
- C the temperature at which the latent heat of vaporisation equals zero
- D -182.5°C for oxygen
- E -118.4°C for oxygen

Your answers: A.......B.......C.......D.......E.......

36 The saturated vapour pressure (SVP) of a liquid

- A depends on the atmospheric pressure
- B depends on its volume
- C depends on its temperature
- D can be expressed in mmHg
- E equals atmospheric pressure at its boiling point

Your answers: A.......B.......C.......D.......E.......

MCQ Exam 2

37 Block of the cervical sympathetic ganglia produces

    A   dilatation of the conjunctival vessels
    B   anhydrosis of the ipsilateral face
    C   miosis
    D   nasal congestion
    E   exophthalmos

Your answers: A.......B.......C.......D.......E.......

38 A complete block of the ulnar nerve at the elbow will lead to

    A   numbness of the ulnar side of the forearm
    B   paralysis of the hypothenar muscles
    C   paralysis of all the thenar muscles
    D   sensory loss over the little finger
    E   sensory loss over the medial side of the ring finger

Your answers: A.......B.......C.......D.......E.......

39 Carbon monoxide

    A   has 150 times greater affinity for haemoglobin than oxygen
    B   stimulates the chemoreceptors
    C   in smokers can combine with up to 15% of the haemoglobin
    D   is rapidly eliminated by breathing high oxygen concentrations
    E   shifts the oxygen dissociation curve to the left

Your answers: A.......B.......C.......D.......E.......

40 An increase in vagal activity results in the following changes in the heart:

    A   a decrease in rate
    B   an increase in contractility
    C   a decrease in the rate of repolarisation of the pacemaker cells
    D   a prolongation of conduction at the AV node
    E   an increased cardiac output

Your answers: A.......B.......C.......D.......E.......

MCQ Exam 2

41 The cerebrospinal fluid

    A has a higher glucose content than plasma
    B has a higher pH than plasma
    C has a higher protein content than plasma
    D has a total volume of approximately 250 ml
    E is secreted from the arachnoid villi

Your answers: A.......B.......C.......D.......E.......

42 Hartmann's solution (compound sodium lactate) contains

    A 5 mmol of potassium per litre
    B calcium chloride
    C more sodium than normal saline
    D magnesium sulphate
    E 150 mmol of chloride per litre

Your answers: A.......B.......C.......D.......E.......

43 The muscles used in active expiration include

    A diaphragm
    B rectus abdominis
    C external oblique
    D internal oblique
    E strap muscles

Your answers: A.......B.......C.......D.......E.......

44 The acute loss of more than 500 ml of blood in the adult results in the following effects:

    A severe vasoconstriction in the cerebral circulation
    B a reduction of the glomerular filtration rate
    C increased aldosterone secretion
    D increased rate of discharge from the arterial baroreceptors
    E reduced ADH production

Your answers: A.......B.......C.......D.......E.......

MCQ Exam 2

45 Cardiac output is increased by

- A a rise in venous filling pressure
- B a rise in body temperature
- C an increased metabolic rate
- D standing up from the lying position
- E pregnancy in the last trimester

Your answers: A.......B.......C.......D.......E.......

46 Cerebral blood flow will be increased by

- A a rise in arterial PCO_2 to 8 kPa (60 mmHg)
- B a head down posture
- C an increase in systemic BP from 110 to 130 mmHg
- D hyperventilation
- E a rise in arterial PO_2

Your answers: A.......B.......C.......D.......E.......

47 Inaccuracies in the measurement of central venous pressure (CVP) may arise from

- A a change in position of the patient
- B misplacement of the catheter
- C wetting of the cotton wool plug in the top of the manometer tube
- D straining during respiration
- E arterial hypotension

Your answers: A.......B.......C.......D.......E.......

48 In the normal heart

- A blood in the left atrium contains less oxygen than blood in the pulmonary artery
- B right ventricular pressure might be 25/10 mmHg
- C pulmonary artery systolic pressure is usually about 10 mmHg less than right ventricular systolic pressure
- D left ventricular pressure might be 125/3 mmHg
- E blood in the pulmonary artery has an oxygen saturation of 75%

Your answers: A.......B.......C.......D.......E.......

MCQ Exam 2

49 Transmitters at the autonomic ganglia include

    A   5-HT
    B   glycine
    C   acetylcholine
    D   butylcholine
    E   noradrenaline

Your answers: A.......B.......C.......D.......E.......

50 Reabsorption of sodium in the kidney

    A   is regulated by ADH
    B   occurs in the proximal tubule
    C   occurs by active transport in the loop of Henle
    D   is influenced by Starling's forces
    E   is associated with chloride reabsorption

Your answers: A.......B.......C.......D.......E.......

51 Results of prolonged severe vomiting, complicating pyloric stenosis include

    A   hyperchloraemia
    B   impaired renal bicarbonate excretion
    C   hyperventilation
    D   acidic urine excretion
    E   hypokalaemia

Your answers: A.......B.......C.......D.......E.......

52 ABO blood groups

    A   are an example of Mendelian dominant inheritance
    B   may be detected in saliva
    C   are independent of Rhesus blood groups
    D   AB blood can be given to A and B recipients
    E   O negative blood can be given to anyone

Your answers: A.......B.......C.......D.......E.......

MCQ Exam 2

53 In digoxin toxicity

   A   the ECG characteristically shows widespread RST segment depression
   B   intravenous calcium gluconate may temporarily reverse the toxic effects on the myocardium
   C   phenytoin may be helpful in the treatment of supraventricular dysrhythmias
   D   corticosteroids may restore normal conduction if heart block is present
   E   the plasma digoxin level is a reliable guide to severity

Your answers: A.......B.......C.......D.......E.......

54 A longstanding, uncomplicated transection of the spinal cord at the level of C5 results in

   A   flaccid paralysis of the legs
   B   loss of a shivering reflex
   C   loss of a micturition reflex
   D   hyperkalaemia with suxamethonium administration
   E   absence of sweat gland activity below the level of the lesion

Your answers: A.......B.......C.......D.......E.......

55 ECG changes in hyperkalaemia include

   A   prominent P waves
   B   prominent T waves
   C   prominent U waves
   D   increased QRS duration
   E   a shortened PR interval

Your answers: A.......B.......C.......D.......E.......

56 Postoperative urinary retention in women is commonly caused by

   A   spinal anaesthesia
   B   fluid overload
   C   neostigmine
   D   morphine
   E   perineal operations

Your answers: A.......B.......C.......D.......E.......

MCQ Exam 2

57 Compared with fresh blood, citrate phosphate dextrose (CPD) blood stored for 21 days contains

    A   as many functioning platelets
    B   increased extracellular potassium
    C   increased lactate
    D   normal 2,3-diphosphoglycerate levels
    E   more extracellular haemoglobin

Your answers: A.......B.......C.......D.......E.......

58 A shift to the right of the trachea usually occurs with

    A   diffuse emphysema of the left lung
    B   a right sided nodular goitre
    C   right pneumothorax
    D   left pneumonectomy
    E   left sided lung collapse

Your answers: A.......B.......C.......D.......E.......

59 A chronic bronchitic who normally has an arterial PCO_2 of 8.0 kPa (60 mmHg) and an arterial PO_2 of 8.0 kPa is found to have the following arterial blood gases:- pH 7.29, PCO_2 8.26 kPa (62 mmHg), PO_2 8.13 kPa (61 mmHg), HCO_2 29.6 mmol/l, BE +0.5, SBC 24.5 mmol/l

    A   he has an acidosis due to recent worsening of his bronchitis (acute on chronic)
    B   he has developed metabolic acidosis
    C   he could not have a metabolic acidosis with a BE of +0.5
    D   these are normal blood gases for him
    E   he has metabolic and respiratory alkalosis

Your answers: A.......B.......C.......D.......E.......

60 An abnormal response to a Valsalva manoeuvre may occur with

    A   hypertension
    B   heart failure
    C   adrenergic blocking drugs
    D   myasthenia gravis
    E   diabetic autonomic neuropathy

Your answers: A.......B.......C.......D.......E.......

END OF PRACTICE EXAM 2

Go over your answers until your time is up.
Answers and explanations are on page 105.

THE WRITTEN PAPER

The Regulations state
"Unlike the MCQ, the essay questions are not designed solely to test accurate recall of facts: a good essay answer contains indications of the candidate's ability to select the most relevant pieces of information, to assign relative importance to them and to assemble a logically inter-related dissertation or argument. Tabulated, telegraphic answers in which all the correct information is randomly located within material that is of doubtful relevance are not, therefore, of a pass standard.

The essays are also a test of the candidate's ability to communicate clearly and unambiguously and thus legibility and a reasonable command of the English language are of relevance.

The essay paper will contain 7 questions which are all compulsory. Candidates should not assume that they are necessarily all of equal weight".

DISTRIBUTION OF QUESTIONS
The balance of questions that can be expected is

1. Anatomy, often includes a local anaesthetic block
2. Medicine or surgery
3. Therapeutics, usually pharmacology of anaesthetic drugs
4. 'Physics', anaesthetic apparatus and monitoring
5. Physiology
6 and 7. Anaesthetic clinical practice

Short note questions with three separate parts have been included.

DOING THE PAPER
The general advice for written papers is straightforward. Read the questions carefully a number of times. Underline the key words. Start listing the topics you intend to include in your answer. Begin writing with a question you feel confident about to get in the correct frame of mind. Do not spend more than the right proportion of time on any one question. Keep asking yourself *'Am I answering the question?'* In an anaesthetic exam always consider if the question could include local as well as general anaesthesia. Keep adding to your list of topics for the questions you are less sure about, often things will come to mind as you are answering other questions. Read through your answers.

Essays should be essays not lists. 'Discuss' should contain discussion and comparison. 'Anaesthetic management' means everything an anaesthetist would be expected to do. ' Operative management ' means the anaes-

The Written Paper

thetist's management in the operating theatre. Diagrams can be used but be sure they are well drawn and labelled. Lists are best used only if time is desperately short. Selective underlining can be helpful but should not be overdone. Keep sentences short and do not include more than 2 or 3 points in each paragraph.

In relation to the Part 1 examination it is essential to appreciate that with 7 questions, all of which must be answered and the use of close marking, a uniform standard of answers is required, one bad answer is almost certain to wreck the candidates chances however good the other questions may be. 20-25 minutes is the maximum time that should be allowed for writing on any one question if sufficient time is to be allowed for planning answers and reading through at the end.

It is important to note the remarks in the Regulations concerning legibility and command of the English language. Bad spelling always irritates the examiner and poor writing wastes his time which is worse. It is usually better to write less and make sure that it is easy to read. If the writing is illegible the paper is sent to other examiners, if they too cannot read it the candidate fails.

Three Written Papers are set out in this section. It is suggested that you should do the Written Papers in as close to examination conditions as possible. Outline answers are provided later in the book to help to ensure that your factual content is complete but you are advised to show your answers to more senior colleagues to gain their opinion, particularly with regard to your layout and style.

WRITTEN PAPER 1

Time allowed 3 hours.

Candidates MUST answer ALL questions and are advised that the omission of any question is likely to result in failure to pass the paper.

1. Describe the anatomical structures encountered in the passage of a needle for spinal anaesthesia.

2. Describe the physiological effects of passive hyperventilation.

3. A patient with chronic bronchitis is to have a general anaesthetic, what tests of respiratory function would be of value and what would be the significance of the results obtained?

4. What are the actions of intravenous barbiturates on the cardiovascular system? Discuss briefly their clinical significance.

5. What are the indications for awake intubation in the adult? Describe the local anaesthetic technique that you would use for this procedure.

6. Describe your anaesthetic management of a 25 year old woman, who is 35 weeks pregnant and has developed appendicitis.

7. Discuss the causes and treatment of a sudden rise in blood pressure during general anaesthesia for a laparotomy.

WRITTEN PAPER 2

Time allowed 3 hours.

Candidates MUST answer ALL questions and are advised that the omission of any question is likely to result in failure to pass the paper.

1. Describe the anatomical structures below the epiglottis seen during bronchoscopy.

2. Describe the physiological mechanisms by which arterial hypoxaemia may occur.

3. Describe briefly the physical principles involved in the functioning of calibrated anaesthetic vaporisers.

4. Compare and contrast the pharmacological effects of vecuronium and d- tubocurarine.

5. Describe in detail the management of intravenous regional anaesthesia (Bier's block) in the upper limb.

6. A woman in shock is thought to have an ectopic pregnancy, describe briefly your anaesthetic management.

7. How may hypercarbia develop during anaesthesia, what clinical changes may result?

WRITTEN PAPER 3

Time allowed 3 hours.

Candidates MUST answer ALL questions and are advised that the omission of any question is likely to result in failure to pass the paper.

1. Describe the relations of the internal jugular vein, what are the common complications of internal jugular cannulation.

2. Compare the physiological response to the infusion of 1 litre of normal saline with that resulting from the infusion of 1 litre of plasma.

3. Describe the Mapleson classification for anaesthetic circuits indicating to which group the circuits in common use belong.

4. What is the safe maximum dose of the commonly used local anaesthetic drugs? What may occur clinically with overdosage?

5. Discuss the advantages and disadvantages of spinal and general anaesthesia for a patient requiring surgery for a fractured neck of femur.

6. Discuss the problems posed for the anaesthetist by patients with narcotic addiction.

7. What action would you take when you find yourself unexpectedly unable to intubate a patient at emergency Caesarean section.

THE ORALS

Vivas probably engender more nervousness amongst candidates than any other part of the examination. While it is almost impossible to pass a viva with no knowledge, it is quite easy to fail one, despite reasonable knowledge, by poor technique. There are two vivas in this exam: a traditional oral and a clinical oral.

The Oral
Half an hour with two examiners. There is no doubt that the best antidote to nervousness is a broad base of knowledge: the feeling that whatever you are asked you would at least know something about the subject. Vivas are like climbing a tree. The first question is usually straight forward: the main trunk. One then explores main branches and then small branches, finally (provided you have answered correctly) on to small twigs at which point you fall off. The only thing candidates remember is the obscure twig they fell off. They do not remember that in getting there they answered many more important things correctly.

The examiner is trying to get an idea of the breadth of your knowledge and once he sees that you know about a topic will switch, often abruptly, to another. Candidates often comment afterwards on the amount of ground covered. It is tempting to try and spin out one topic if you know about it for fear of being asked something you do not know. This is usually a mistake. The more knowledge you can display on different topics the better.

We have not attempted to give practice vivas in this book, but here are a few hints on preparing yourself.

Practice
Get your consultant to give you a few practice vivas, so that you can improve your technique and build up confidence. Many candidates fail to do themselves justice through nervousness and unfamiliarity. Try to relax and speak audibly. Think before blurting out the first thing that comes into your head. Always start with common things. Remember that any anaesthetic starts with a preoperative visit. If asked how to manage an asthmatic for a vaginal hysterectomy, do not leap in with an epidural before assessing the patient.

Listen to the question
It is very irritating for examiners if you answer a question you were not asked. If asked "How would you anaesthetise a fit young man for a hernia", say what you usually do. If on the other hand the question is "What are the possible techniques of anaesthesia for herniorrhaphy" list the different techniques, do not say "My consultant always paralyses and ventilates them".

The Orals

Leading the examiner or digging a pit
Most of the time the examiner leads the candidate. You may be able to lead the examiner, but there is a fine distinction between leading to things you know about and leading to the edge of a bottomless pit which you may be pushed into. Unless you are a very good candidate it is probably better to let the examiner do the leading and try and steer away from pits. Remember that questions often follow on from the previous answer so it is foolish to volunteer that you would estimate the shunt from the shunt equation if you do not know the shunt equation. Untruths are usually obvious as the following exchange shows. "What was the last anaesthetic you gave?" "D & C" "What about the one before that?" "D & C" "Don't you do any other procedures?" "I only do D&C's" Even if this were true, such a candidate would be unlikely to impress the examiners.

Equipment
There are lots of pieces of equipment around as a starting point for discussion e.g. spinal needles, ventimasks, various tubes, anaesthetic machines. If you do not know its name at least describe what it is for. Physics of equipment is asked: it is surprising how many people do not know the pressures at various points in an anaesthetic machine. Do not be surprised if you are asked to draw diagrams to illustrate points.

Long silences
You are not scoring any points when silent. Many examiners think of answers and then design questions to get that answer from the candidate. You may go round and round in circles without seeing what point is being sought. In these circumstances it is probably best to say you do not see what he is getting at, in the hope of moving on to something you do know about.

The Clinical Oral
In this part of the exam candidates are given 10 minutes on their own to study clinical material (there are no actual patients). This usually consists of history, examination findings and results of, for example, chest X-ray, ECG, pulmonary function tests, blood gases, biochemistry etc. Paper and pencil are provided for making notes while you study this. You then have 20-25 minutes with a pair of examiners who discuss the case and its anaesthetic implications with you. To ensure uniformity each batch of candidates studies the same material and the examiners have a series of guided questions which they may or may not stick to. If discussion of the main case does not fill the 25 minutes, there may be a supplementary topic introduced, again the same for each batch of candidates.

In the following section you are given case histories and results to study followed by questions. The best way to use it is to get a colleague to ask the

The Orals

questions and not to look at the answers until you have had a reasonable discussion of the problems raised. Most of the cases have a number of different problems to think about some are 'single problem' cases such as might be asked as a supplementary.

Case Histories

CASE HISTORY 1

A 51 year old advertising executive presents for extraction of his wisdom teeth.

History
He has not attended his doctor for many years and is on no medication.

Examination and Investigations
On admission to the ward his blood pressure is found to be 170/110 and he weighs 80 kg. A chest X-ray (Fig 1) and ECG (Fig 2) are performed.

Anaesthesia
After premedication with papaveretum 20 mg and hyoscine 0.4 mg anaesthesia is induced with thiopentone, the nasal mucosa sprayed with cocaine 10% 2 ml, and a nasotracheal tube is passed with the patient breathing spontaneously nitrous oxide, oxygen and halothane with 7% CO_2 to induce hyperventilation. A throat pack is inserted and the patient breathes N_2O 4 l/min:O_2 2 l/min, halothane 2% via a Bain circuit. During extraction of the teeth his BP rises to 200/115 and his ECG changes as shown (Fig 3).

Questions

1. Comment on his blood pressure on admission. How would you check on this reading?

2. Comment on the chest X-ray and ECG.

3. What should have been done before this patient was anaesthetised?

4. Was the method of induction appropriate for this patient?

5. What fresh gas flow would you have used for maintenance?

6. Comment on the operative ECG.

7. List possible causes for the rising BP and ECG abnormality.

CASE HISTORY 2

History
A 63 year old diabetic lady who lives alone is admitted to hospital with a history of being confused for two days, vomiting for 3 hours and pain in the right leg. Her diabetes is normally controlled on diet and chlorpropamide 250 mg daily. She also has angina for which she takes propranolol 40 mg tds and sublingual glyceryl trinitrate when required.

Examination
Her right foot is found to be gangrenous and a below knee amputation is proposed. She is barely conscious with a pulse of 113, BP 95/65 and weight 58 kg.

Investigations on admission are as follows:

WBC	11.7	$\times 10^9/l$	Plasma sodium	152	mmol/l
RBC	5.19	$\times 10^{12}/l$	potassium	5.3	mmol/l
Hb	15.1	g/dl	chloride	119	mmol/l
Hct	0.48		urea	25	mmol/l
MCV	92	fl	Serum albumin	57	g/l
MCH	29.1	Pg	Blood glucose	34.3	mmol/l
MCHC	31.4	g/dl	Urine glucose	2%	
			Urine ketones	neg	

Arterial blood gases breathing air:

pH	7.34
PCO_2	4.93 kPa (37 mmHg)
PO_2	10.9 kPa (81 mmHg)
HCO_3	19.8 mmol/l
TCO_2	20.8 mmol/l
BE	−5.1 mmol/l
SBC	18.8 mmol/l

Questions

1. Comment on the investigations and describe her metabolic state.

2. Estimate a) the plasma osmolality
   b) the change in her extracellular fluid volume.

3. How soon after admission should surgery go ahead?

4. How would you manage this patient before and during anaesthesia?

5. Briefly describe how you would manage the diabetes of this patient had she come in well controlled for elective minor surgery.

Case Histories

CASE HISTORY 3

An obese man aged 40 needs surgery for repair of an inguinal hernia.

History
He has always been obese. He has pains in the chest after meals and on severe exertion (which is rare for him).

Examination
Height 170 cm. Weight 100 kg.
Pulse 65/min. BP 150/90. No added heart sounds.

Investigations

Chest X-ray (Fig 4)
ECG (Fig 5)

Na	138 mmol/l	Bilirubin	9 mmol/l
K	4.3 mmol/l	Albumin	42 g/l
Cl	102 mmol/l	AST	24 iu/l
Urea	4.4 mmol/l	Alk phos	150 iu/l

Questions

1. Comment on the preoperative investigations.

2. Would you like any further investigations?

3. How much is he over his ideal weight?

4. List the main problems of the obese undergoing surgery.

5. What would be the major risk of giving this patient a general anaesthetic?

6. How could one anaesthetise this patient?

CASE HISTORY 4

History
A 69 year old female is scheduled for repair of a large incisional hernia, which has developed following a sigmoid colectomy for diverticulitis 2 years ago and closure of colostomy one year ago.

She gives an 8 year history of asthma and is also a mild hypertensive. She is on the following drugs:

Salbutamol and beclomethasone (Becotide) inhalers, 2 puffs up to 5 times daily, Moduretic 2 tablets daily, theophylline 400 mg nocte, prednisolone 7.5 mg mane. Nitrazepam, lorazepam, Normacol and Isogel were also in her collection of tablets.

Examination
Pulse 90/min. Blood pressure 140/90. Resps 16/min.

Respiratory function tests

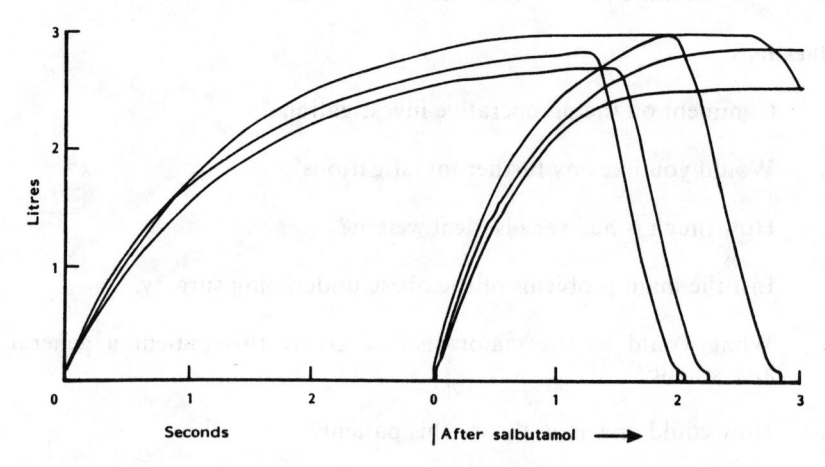

Vitalograph (3 attempts) before and after salbutamol

		% Predicted	after salbutamol
Peak expiratory flow rate	250 l/min	66%	345
FEV_1	1.7 l	61%	2.4
VC	3.0 l	80%	3.0
FEV_1/VC	56%		

Case Histories

Blood gases (breathing air) taken by the house surgeon from a femoral stab were:

pH	7.35		
PCO$_2$	6.13	kPa	(46 mmHg)
PO$_2$	5.60	kPa	(42 mmHg)
HCO$_3$	26.0	mmol/l	
TCO$_2$	27.3	mmol/l	
BE	+0.5	mmol/l	
SBC	25.1	mmol/l	

When repeated by the anaesthetist from a radial artery stab they were:

pH	7.42		
PCO$_2$	5.07	kPa	(38 mmHg)
PO$_2$	10.7	kPa	(80 mmHg)
HCO$_2$	24.4	mmol/l	
TCO$_2$	25.5	mmol/l	
BE	0	mmol/l	
SBC	24.5	mmol/l	

Questions

1. How do you interpret the pulmonary function tests?
2. How do you interpret the blood gases?
3. Would you require any further investigations?
4. How would you anaesthetise this patient?
5. What premedication would you choose?

Case Histories

CASE HISTORY 5

A 79 year old man weighing 63 kg is to undergo transurethral resection of his prostate. He was admitted with acute retention 2 days previously when he was catheterised. At that time his electrolytes were:

Na	138	mmol/l
K	4.9	mmol/l
Cl	104	mmol/l
Urea	8.2	mmol/l

On the morning of the operation they are:

Na	142	mmol/l
K	4.5	mmol/l
Cl	102	mmol/l
Urea	5.8	mmol/l

His ECG is shown (Fig 7)

After premedication with oral diazepam 5 mg he is given a spinal anaesthetic with heavy cinchocaine 0.5% (Nupercain) 2 ml which gives satisfactory anaesthesia up to T8. Transurethral resection is performed by the surgical registrar using glycine 1.5% as the irrigating solution. The operation proves to be difficult: 25 g of prostate are resected, there is troublesome bleeding and the procedure takes 1 1/2 hours. Towards the end the patient becomes confused and disorientated and becomes even more confused and dyspnoeic in recovery. His anaesthetic record is shown. (Fig 8)

Electrolytes taken in recovery are:

Na	118	mmol/l
K	3.5	mmol/l
Cl	85	mmol/l
Urea	3.5	mmol/l

His haematocrit is 32%

Case Histories

Arterial blood gases (breathing O_2 4 l/min by MC mask)

pH	7.45	
PCO_2	4.13	kPa (31 mmHg)
PO_2	8.0	kPa (60 mmHg)
HCO_3	21.5	mmol/l
TCO_2	22.5	mmol/l
BE	−2.0	mmol/l
SBC	22.5	mmol/l

Questions

1. Comment on the two sets of preoperative electrolytes.

2. What does his ECG show?

3. Are any special precautions necessary?

4. How do you interpret the changes in systolic BP shown on the anaesthetic record.

5. Why is the patient becoming confused at the end?

6. What would you expect to find on examining the patient's respiratory and cardiovascular systems in recovery? What does the chest X-ray (Fig 9) show?

7. Where should he go from the recovery room? What treatment needs to be started?

Case Histories

CASE HISTORY 6

A 40 year old accountant is admitted to Casualty with severe abdominal pain of sudden onset. The surgeons want to perform a laparotomy within the hour.

History
He has a long history of epigastric pain treated with cimetidine. He has had no previous operations. His brother had to spend some time in an Intensive Care Unit after a straightforward appendicitis.

Examination
Anxious
Pulse 110/min. BP 120/80. Respirations 16/min.
Board-like rigidity of the abdomen. No bowel sounds.

Investigations

Chest X-ray (Fig 10)
WBC   5.2   x 10^9/l
RBC   4.14   x 10^{12}/l
Hb   8.7   g/dl
Hct   0.31
MCV   75   fl
MCH   21   pg
MCHC   28   g/dl

ECG taken at his last outpatient visit is available (Fig 11)

Questions

1. Comment on the chest X-ray.

2. What is the probable diagnosis?

3. Comment on the blood count and ECG.

4. What might the brother's problem have been? List the possibilities.

5. What further questions would you ask about the brother?

6. How might the answers modify your choice of drugs in this case?

7. Would you be prepared to anaesthetise the patient within an hour?

Case Histories

CASE HISTORY 7

A 39 year old lady is scheduled for laparotomy.

History
Lower abdominal swelling noticed over the last few weeks. No previous operations. Otherwise fit, jogs 2 miles every day.

Examination
Weight 50 kg. BP 130/80. Pulse 68/min. No abnormal findings. Chest X-ray shown (Fig 12).

Anaesthesia and Operation
Premedication: papaveretum 15 mg hyoscine 0.3 mg. Thiopentone 375 mg, fentanyl 100 μg, suxamethonium 100 mg. Following intubation, pancuronium 7 mg, fentanyl 100 μg, are given and she is ventilated with nitrous oxide 5 l/min oxygen 3 l/min and halothane 0.5% via a Manley ventilator, of the minute volume divider type. A simple ovarian cyst is removed and the procedure takes 30 minutes. At the end the patient will not breathe spontaneously despite neostigmine 2.5 mg and glycopyrrolate 0.6 mg.

Questions

1. Comment on the chest X-ray.

2. What are the possible causes of the patient's apnoea?

3. How would you distinguish between them?

4. How can they be treated?

CASE HISTORY 8

A 53 year old patient (photographed postoperatively in figures 13 and 14) presents for cataract extraction under general anaesthesia. He has not had an anaesthetic before, is otherwise fit and weighed 60 kg. He is premedicated with papaveretum 15 mg and hyoscine 0.3 mg, induced with thiopentone and paralysed with atracurium 35 mg. On direct laryngoscopy the junior anaesthetist is able to see the tip of the epiglottis but not the cords and is unable to intubate the trachea. It is easy to ventilate by mask but after further attempts at intubation a tear in the pharyngeal mucosa is noted. The procedure is abandoned at this stage. A postoperative neck X-ray is shown in Fig 15.

Questions

1. Would you have anticipated difficulty in intubating this patient?

2. What preoperative features would lead you to expect a difficult intubation?

3. As a junior anaesthetist what would you have done having found yourself unable to intubate?

4. What are the alternative methods of proceeding with the patient at this stage?

5. How and when would you reverse the muscle relaxation? What would you use to assess this?

6. What is shown on the X-ray (Fig 15).

7. If it is essential to intubate what techniques are available for the difficult intubation?

CASE HISTORY 9

A 35 year old man with an enlarged thyroid is to have it removed surgically.

History
Weight has been constant at 58 kg. Past history of hernia repair three years ago. He has been taking Lugol's iodine for 10 days.

Examination
Diffusely enlarged thyroid. No eye signs. Pulse regular 80/min. BP 130/80.

Investigations

Chest X-ray (Fig 16)

			Normal
Na 142	mmol/l	Thyroxine T_4 128 nmol/l	(60-140)
K 3.8	mmol/l	T_3 2.4 nmol/l	(1-3.5)
Ca 2.34	mmol/l	TSH 3.0 mU/l	(<5)
Phosphate	mmol/l		
Albumin 43	g/l		

After premedication with pethidine 50 mg and atropine 0.6 mg IM one hour preoperatively, he is anaesthetised with methohexitone 60 mg, alcuronium 15 mg, pethidine 15 mg and ventilated via an oral endotracheal tube and a Manley ventilator using N_2O 4 l/min, O_2 2 l/min and enflurane 0.4% (see chart Fig 17). Surgical removal of the goitre is difficult and damage to the right recurrent laryngeal nerve is suspected. On the first postoperative day clinical chemistry results are:

Na	139	mmol/l
K	4.0	mmol/l
Ca	2.04	mmol/l
Phosphate	1.62	mmol/l
Albumin	39	g/l

Questions

1. Are the history and investigations consistent with a diagnosis of thyrotoxicosis?

2. What are the abnormalities of thyroid function tests in

   a) hyperthyroidism
   b) hypothyroidism.

Case Histories

3. What is the effect of Lugol's iodine?

4. Comment on the X-ray (Fig 16).

5. What sort of endotracheal tube would you choose?

6. At the point where the anaesthetic record is stopped, what do you think might be happening?

7. What might be seen at laryngoscopy after extubation?

8. What do the tests on the first postoperative day suggest? What signs might be present? What immediate treatment needs to be given?

CASE HISTORY 10

A 22 year old African man is knocked down by a bus and brought unconscious to Casualty where he is intubated. On examination he is unconscious, but responds to painful stimuli in a purposeful manner. Pupils are equal and reacting. There are no localising neurological signs. He also has a Colle's fracture which the orthopaedic surgeons wish to reduce under anaesthesia.

Investigations
Skull X-ray (Figs 18 and 19)
Haemoglobin 12.8 g/l
Sickledex test: positive

Questions

1. Comment on the skull X-rays.

2. What does the Sickledex result tell you?

3. What further tests would you like?

4. What anaesthesia would you choose for the Colle's fracture reduction?

Case Histories

CASE HISTORY 11

A 47 year old Indian man is to have highly selective vagotomy for duodenal ulceration. He speaks no English and details of his past medical history are difficult to elicit, but he was admitted to another hospital 6 weeks ago with pain of some kind and kept in for 10 days. His preoperative ECG is shown (Fig 20).

Questions

1. Comment on the ECG.

2. What does it show?

3. Is he fit for anaesthesia?

4. What are the risks of anaesthesia and surgery in this patient?

CASE HISTORY 12

A patient arrives back in the Intensive Care Unit for elective ventilation following major surgery. On arrival in the unit at 18.15 his arterial blood gases being ventilated with 40% oxygen were:

pH	7.36	
PCO_2	5.5	kPa (41 mmHg)
PO_2	6.7	kPa (50 mmHg)
HCO_3	23.0	mmol/l
TCO_2	24.4	mmol/l
BE	−2.0	mmol/l
SBC	22.3	mmol/l

A portable chest X-ray taken at 18.20 is shown in Fig 21. Subsequent X-rays at 19.00 (Fig 22) and midnight (Fig 23) are also provided.

Questions

1. What is the difference between a portable AP and the usual PA chest X-ray?

2. How do you interpret the blood gases and chest X-ray (Fig 21) taken on arrival in ITU?

3. Comment on the next chest film (19.00 Fig 22). What has been done since the first film. Would you expect an improvement in blood gases?

4. What should be done next?

5. Comment on the final (midnight) X-ray (Fig 23).

CASE HISTORY 13

A 74 year old lady was admitted to the surgical wards for limited resection of a breast lump. She complained of occasional dizzy spells. On examination her pulse was regular, 46 per minute; BP 140/85; JVP 0; and apart from the breast lump, there were no other abnormal findings. Her ECG is shown (Fig 24).

Questions

1. What does the ECG show?

2. Could this explain her dizziness?

3. How can she be treated?

4. Should this be done before anaesthesia?

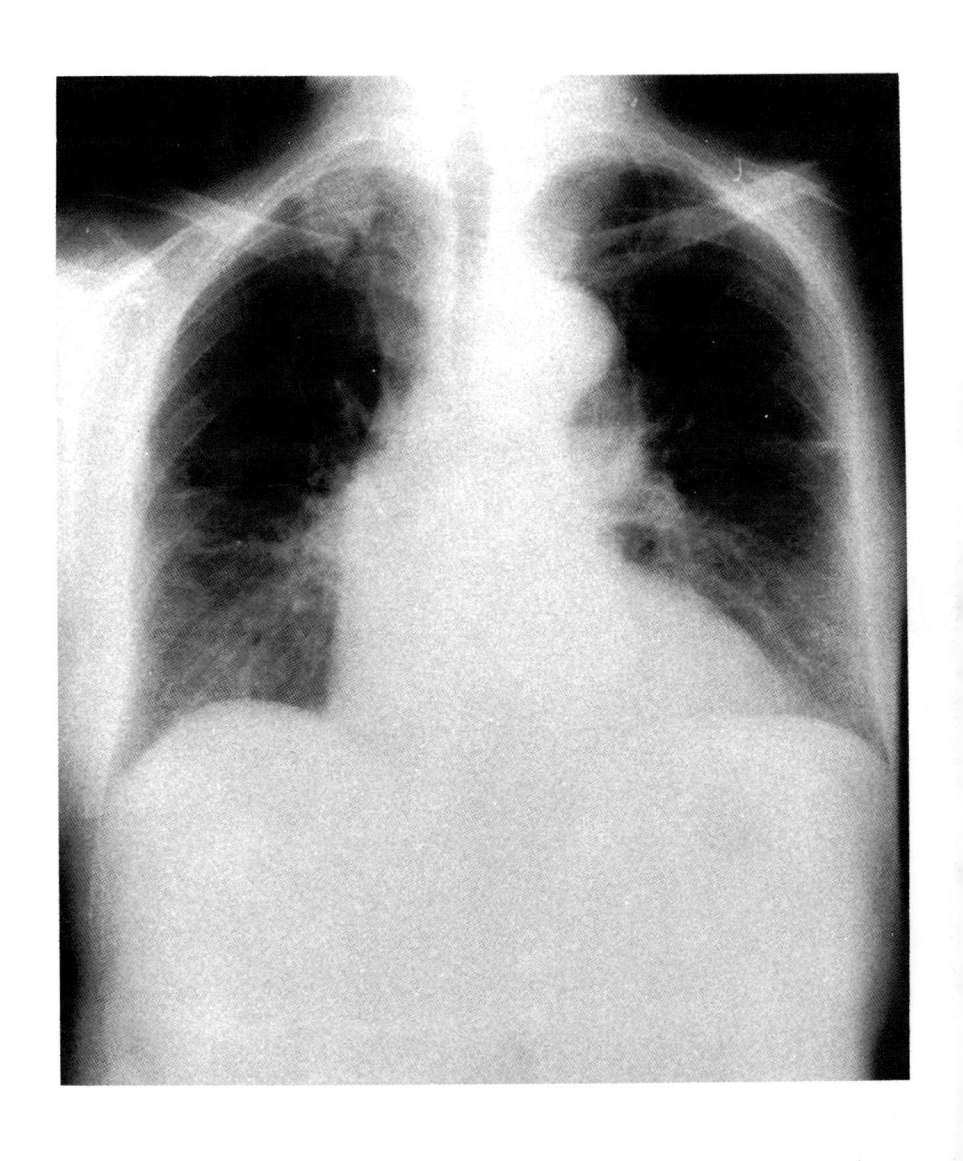

Fig 1. Case 1.

Fig 2. Case 1.

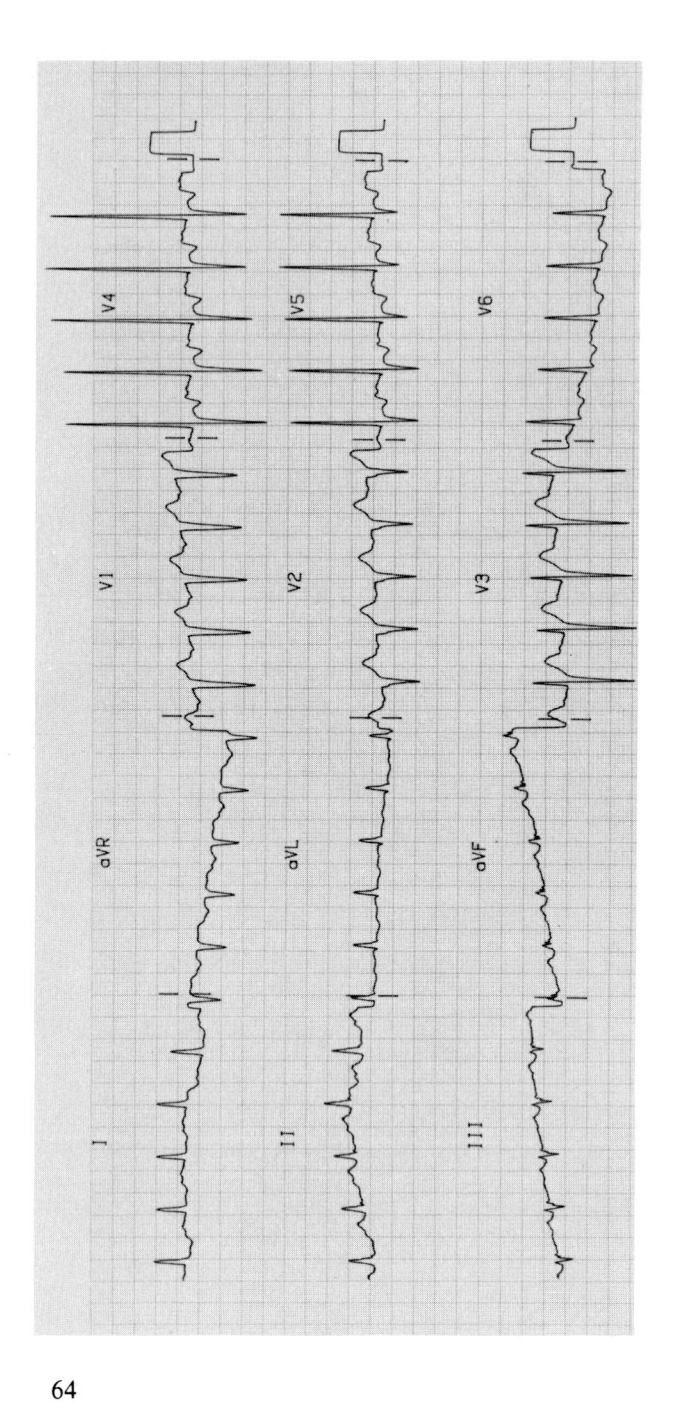

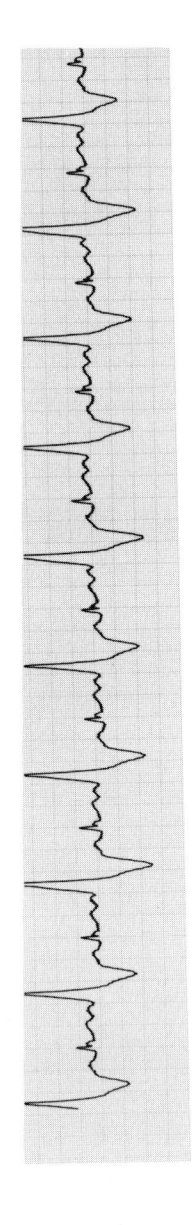

Fig 3. Case 1.

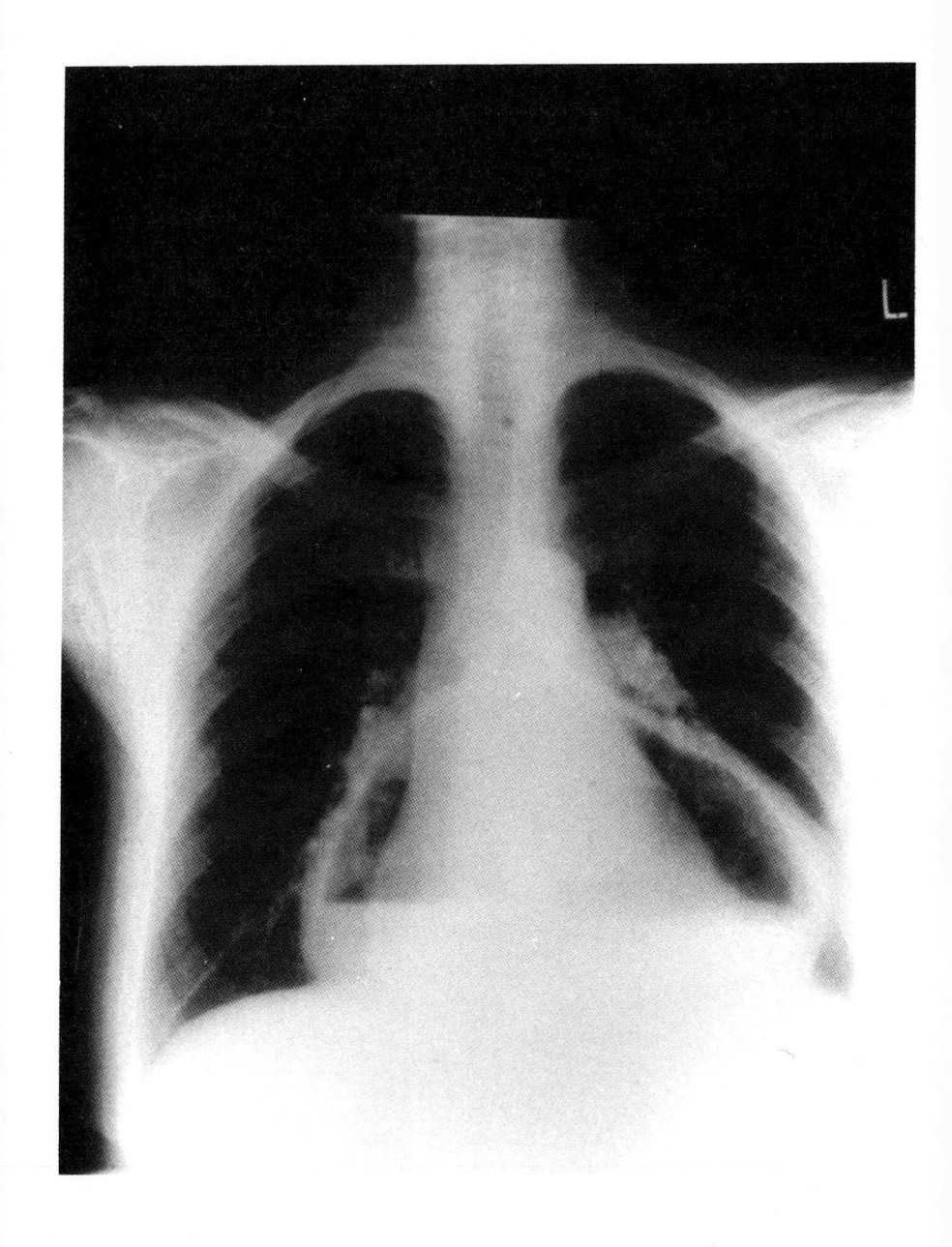

Fig 4. Case 3.

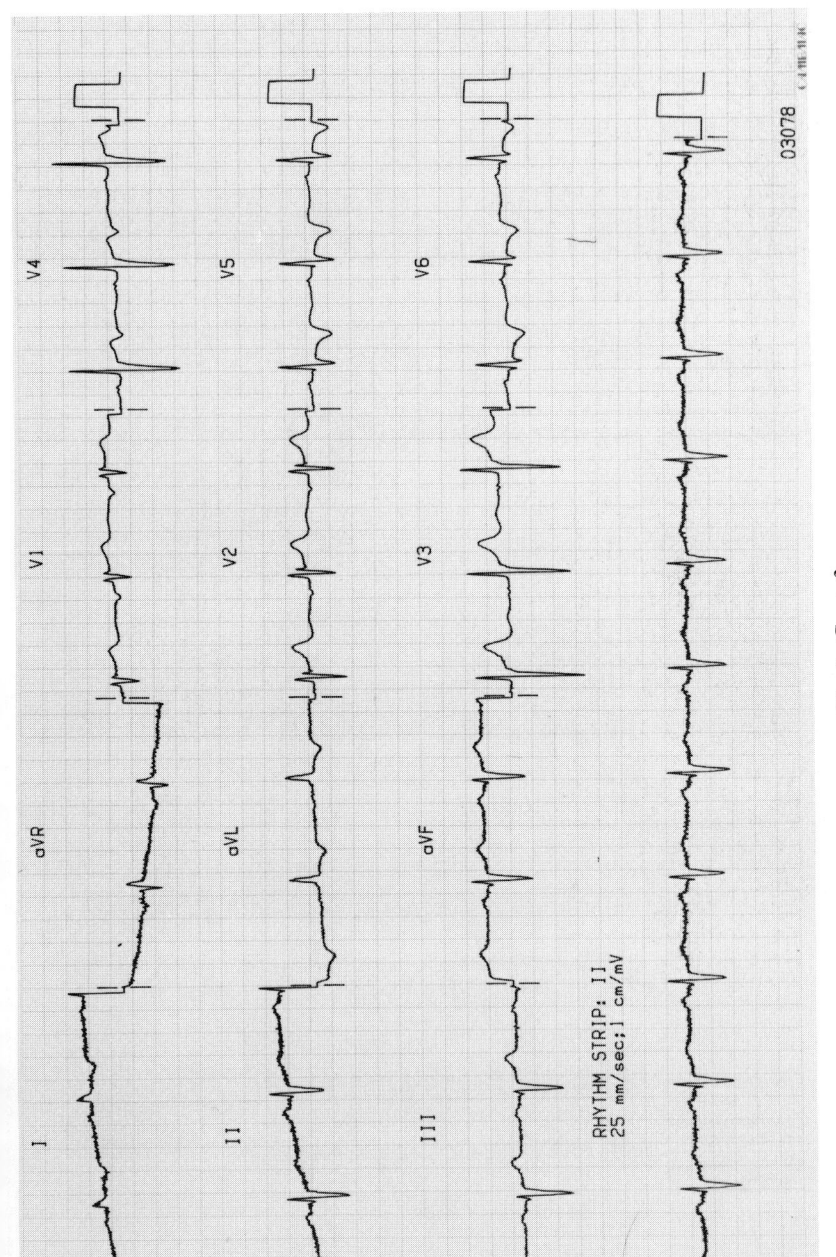

Fig 5. Case 3.

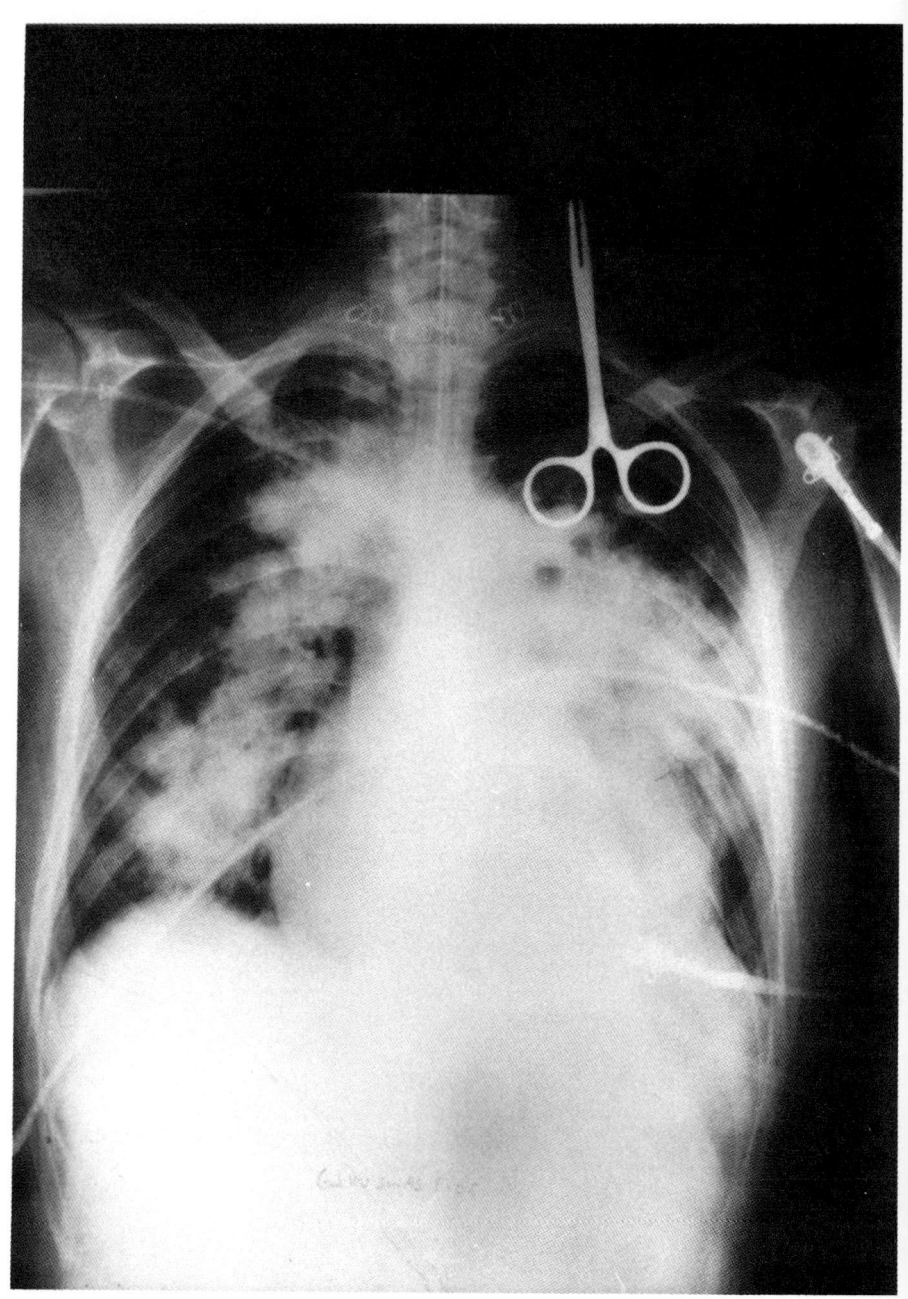

Fig 6. Case 3.

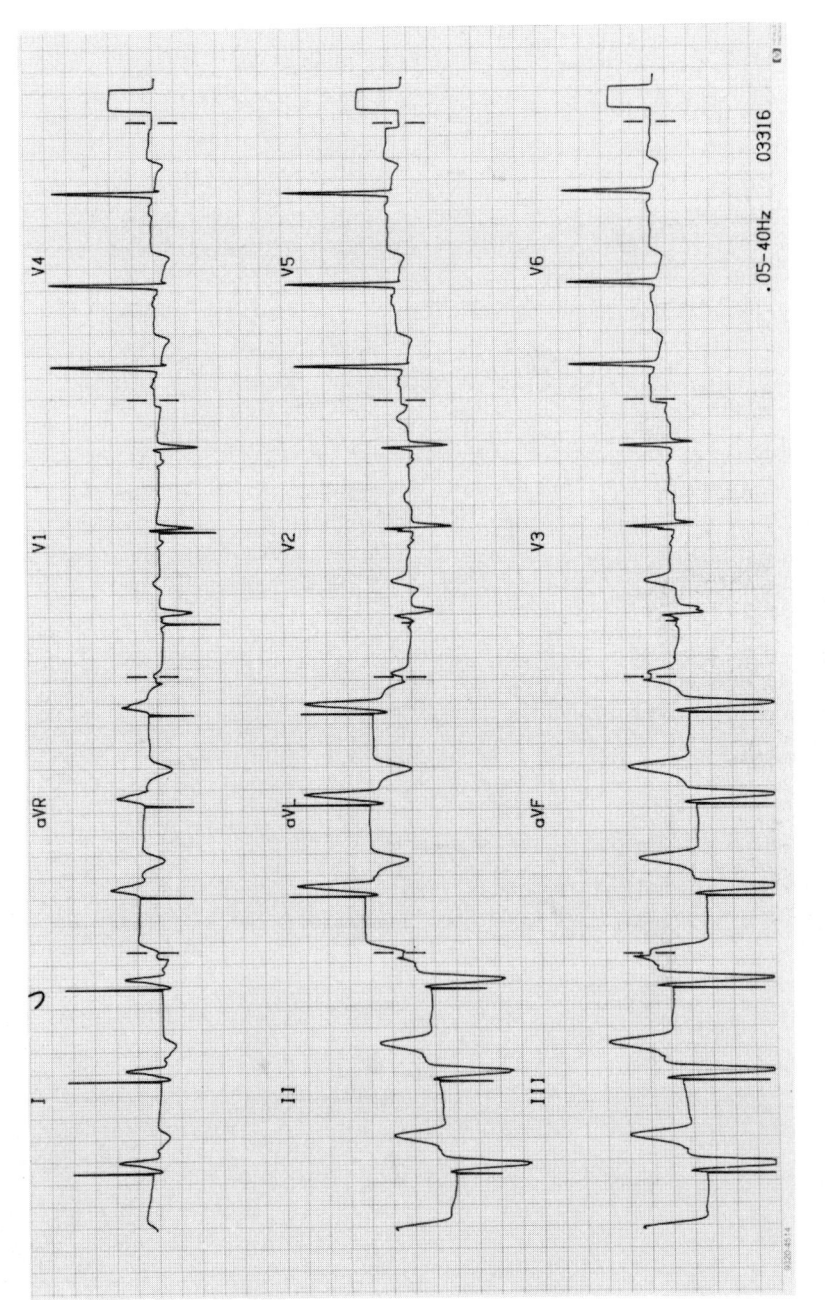

Fig 7. Case 5.

Fig 8. Case 5.

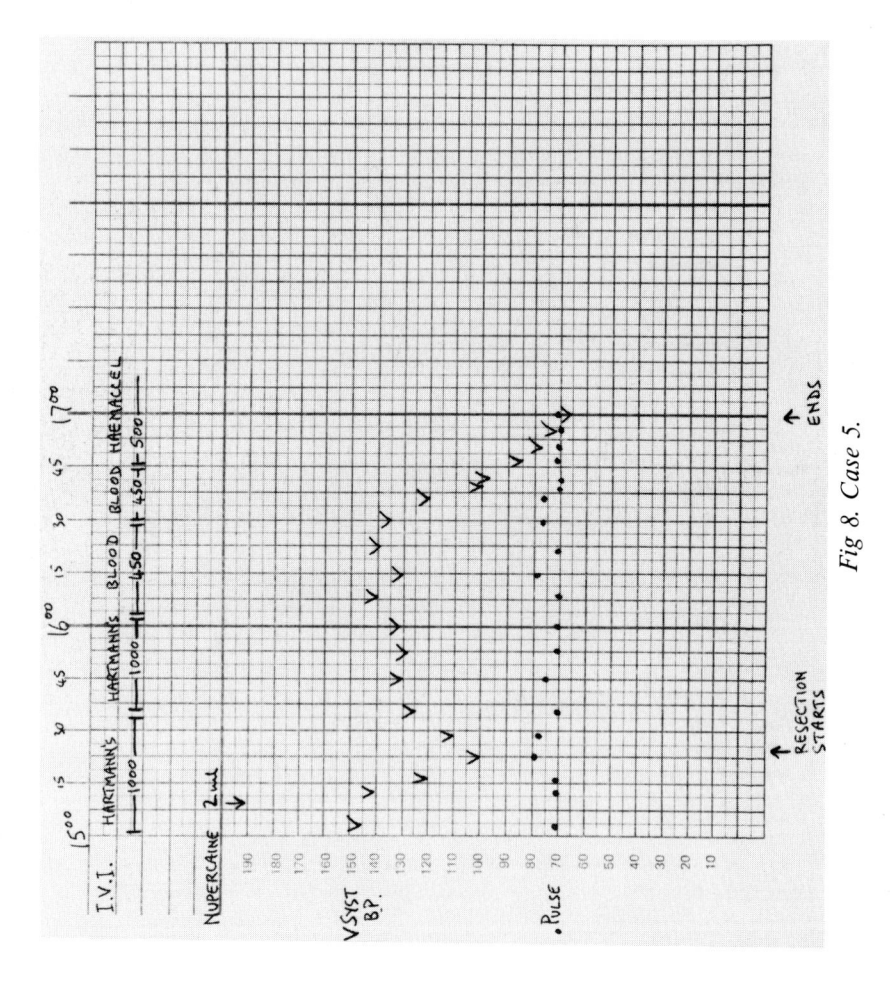

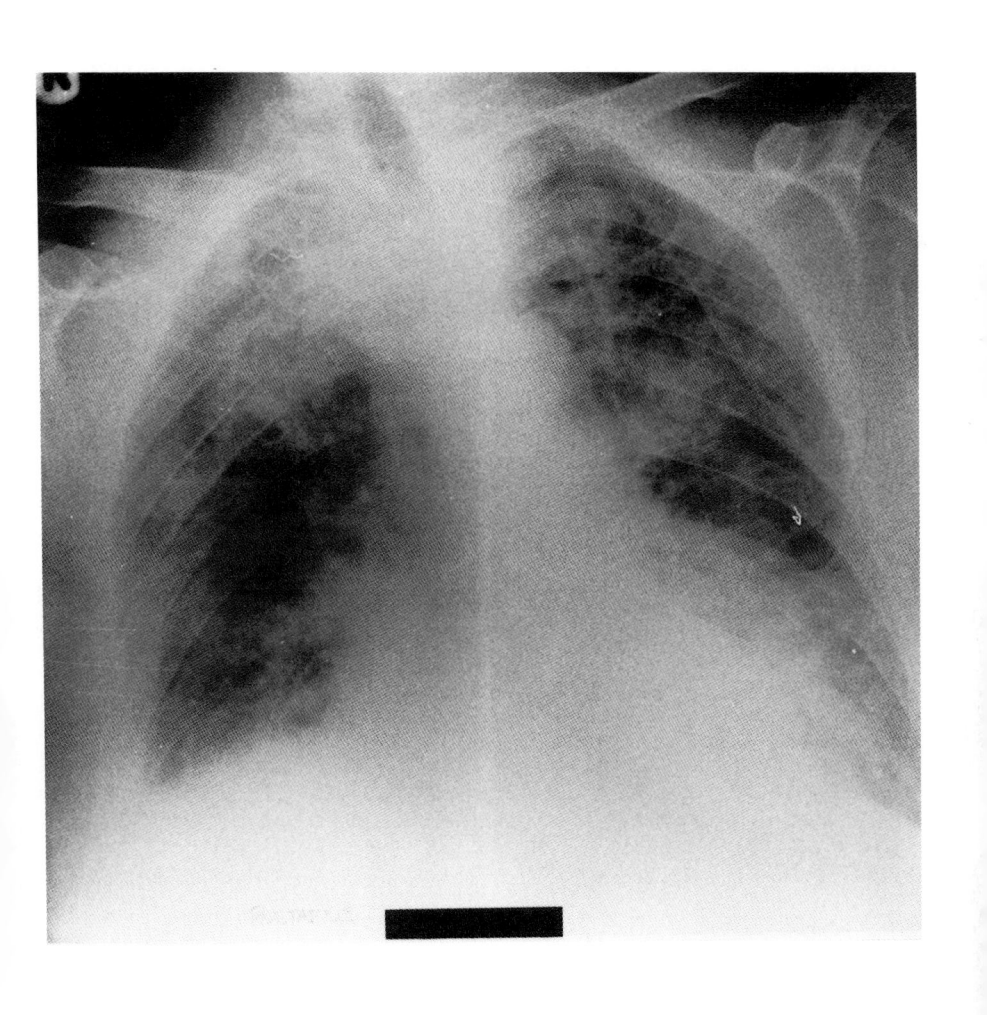

Fig 9. Case 5.

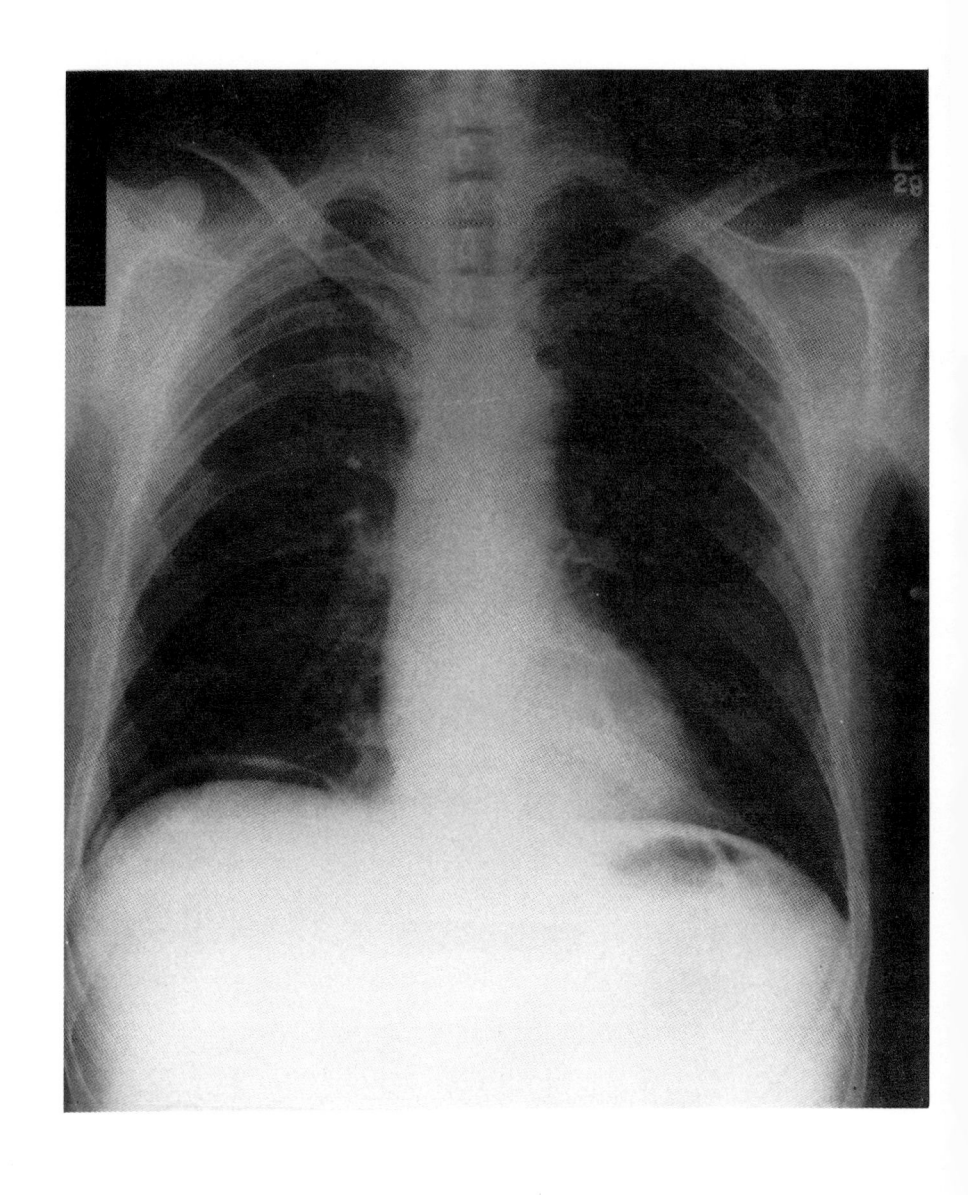

Fig 10. Case 6.

Fig 11. Case 6.

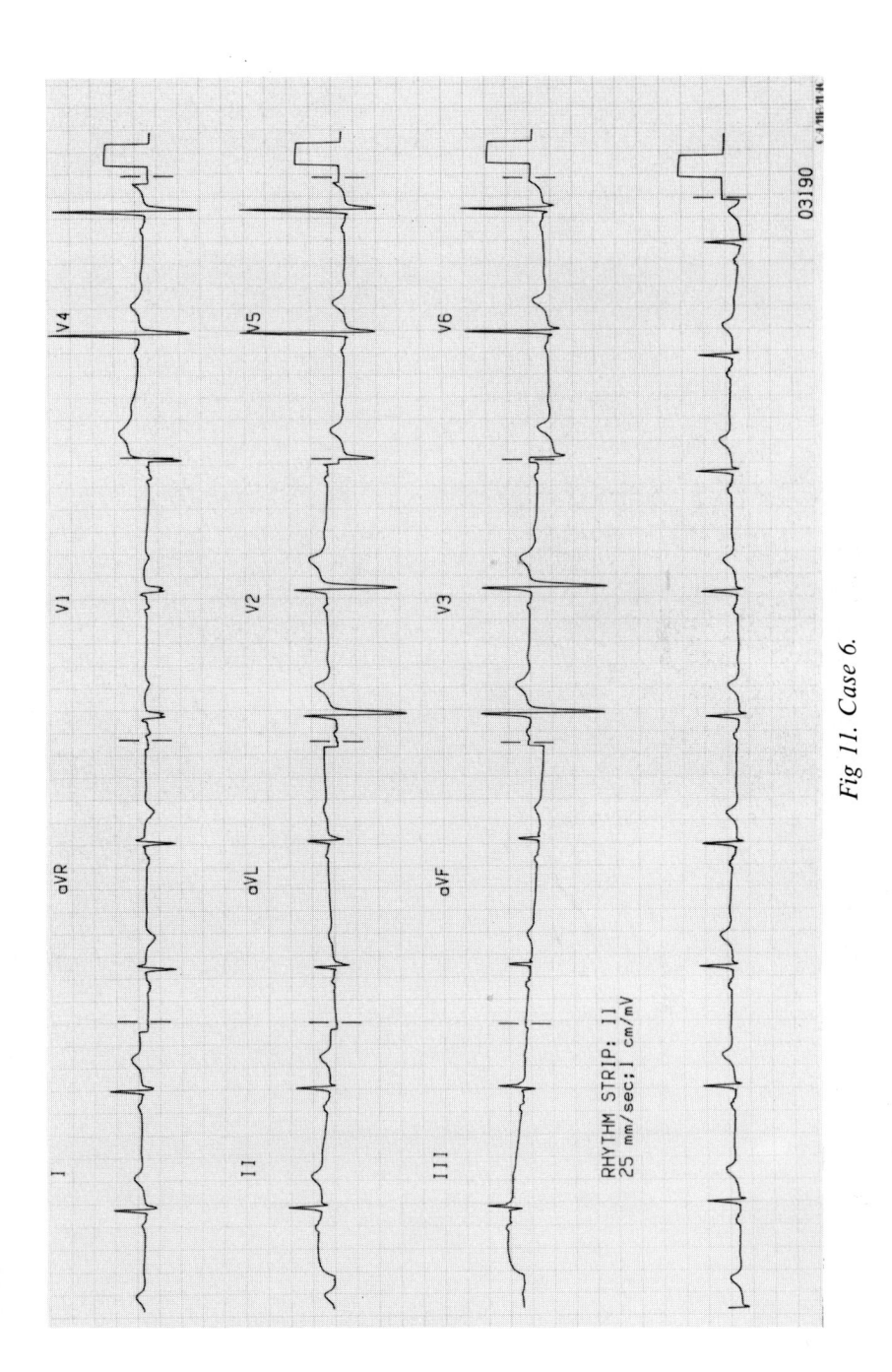

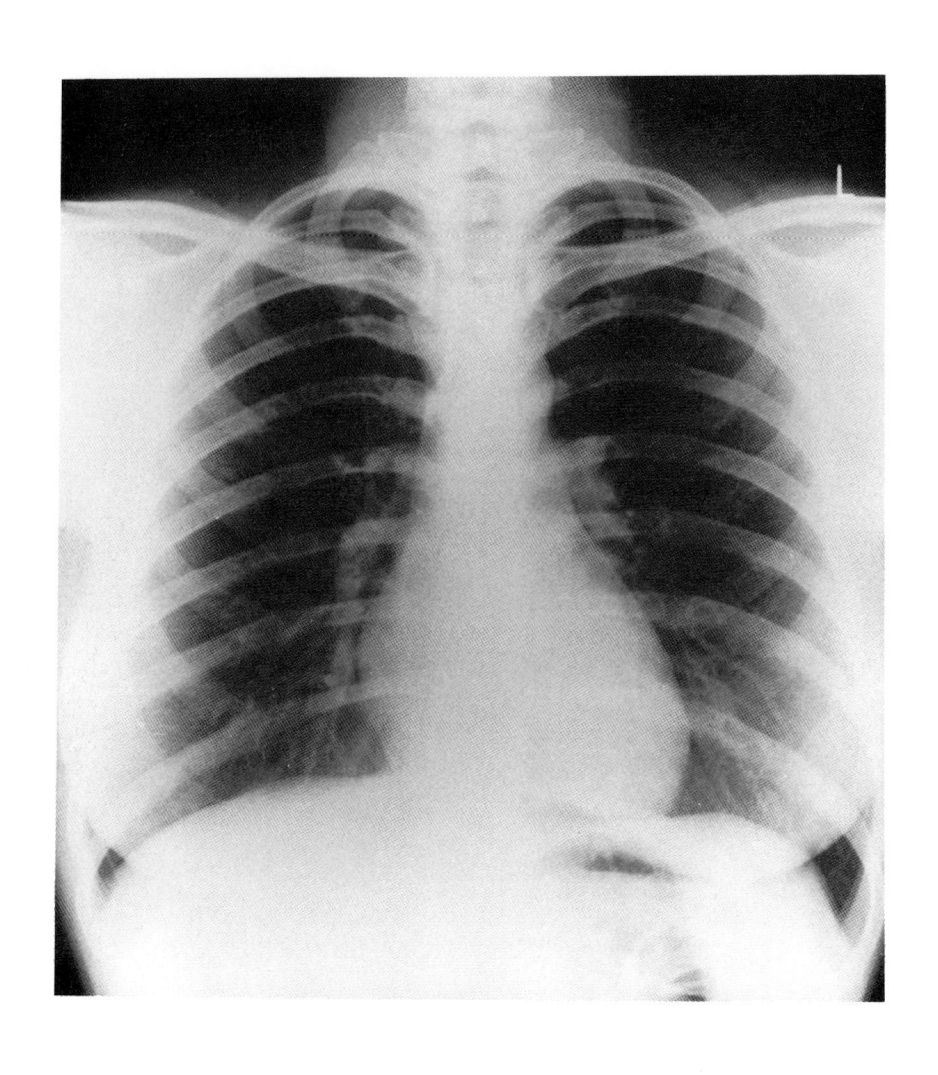

Fig 12. Case 7.

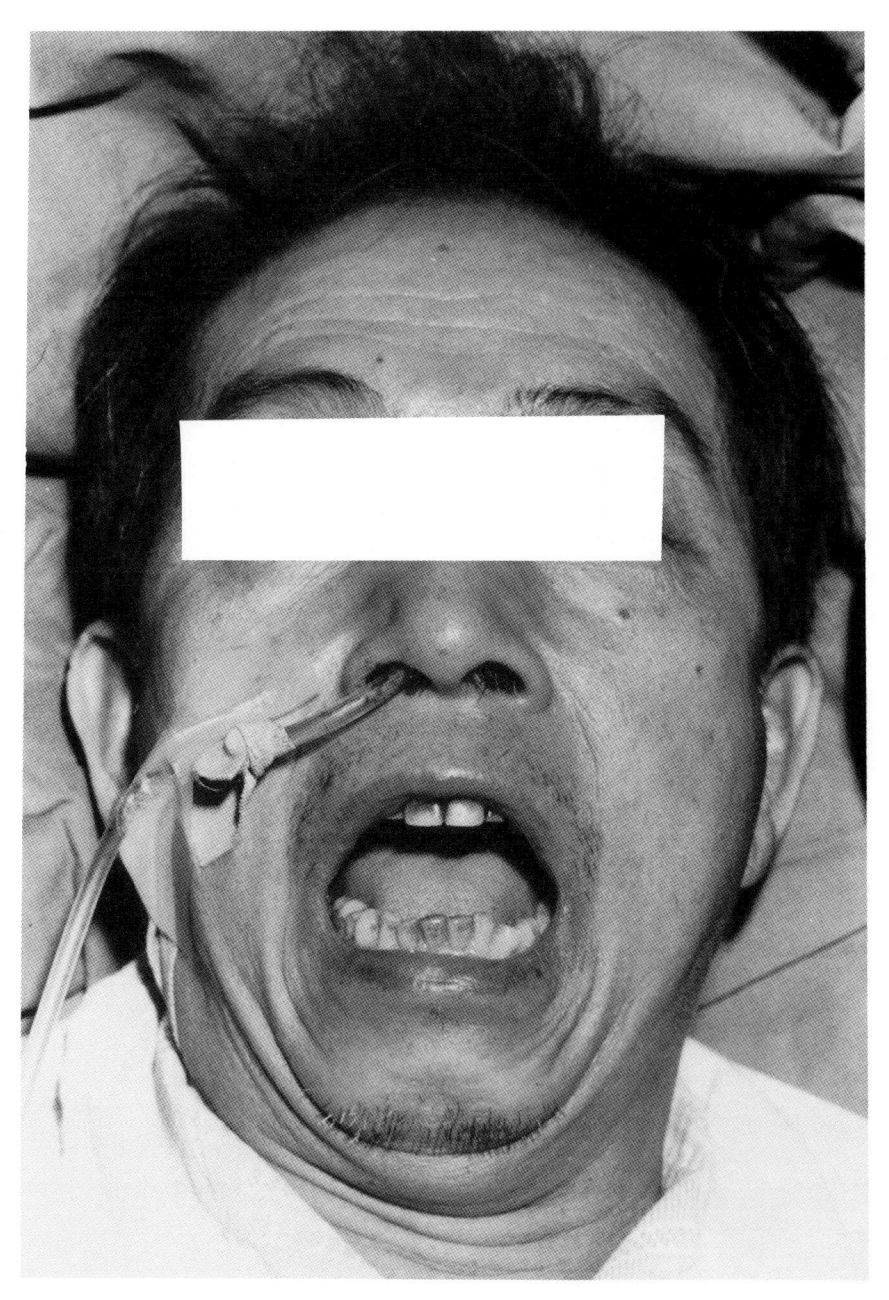

Fig 13. Case 8.

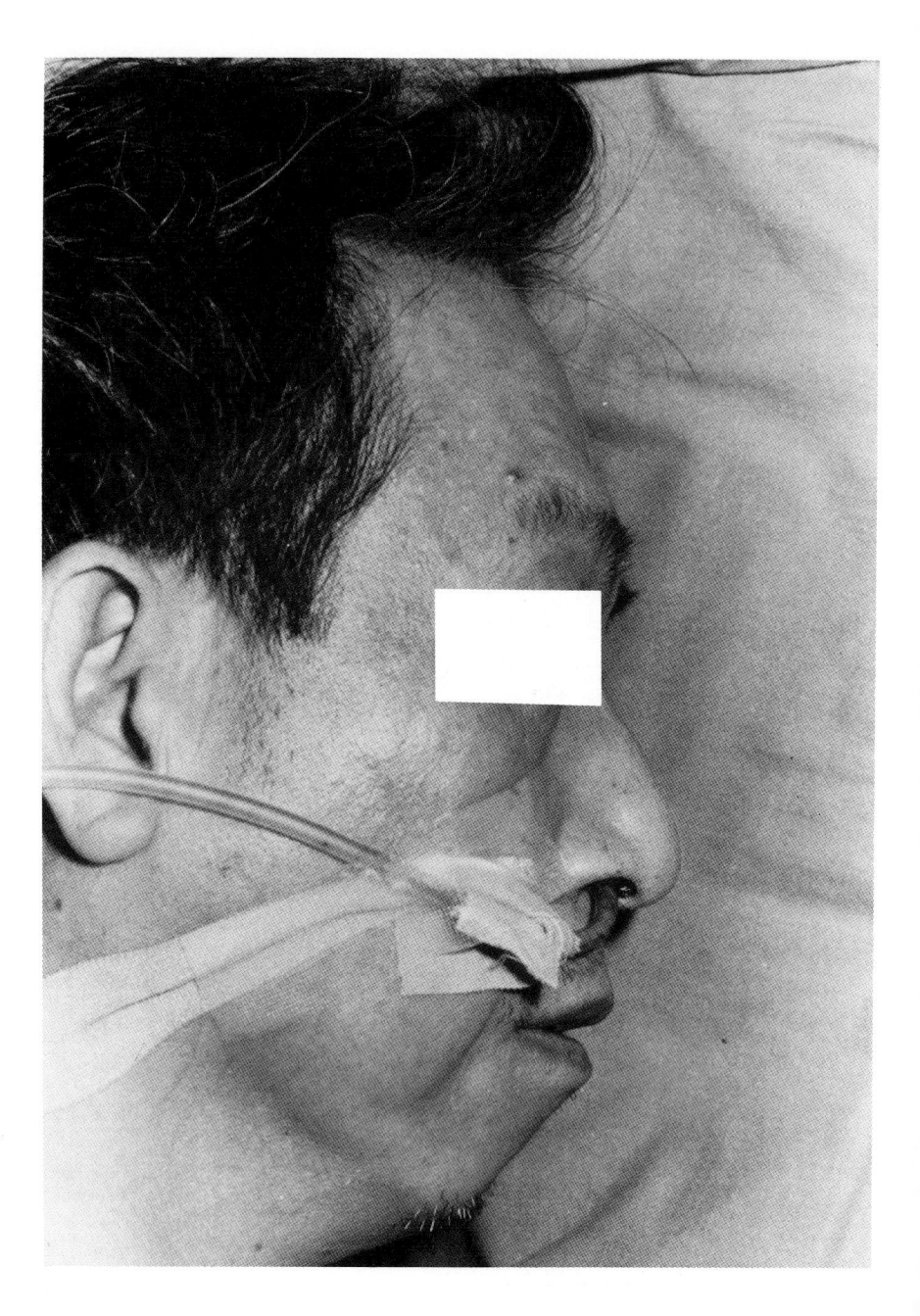

Fig 14. Case 8.

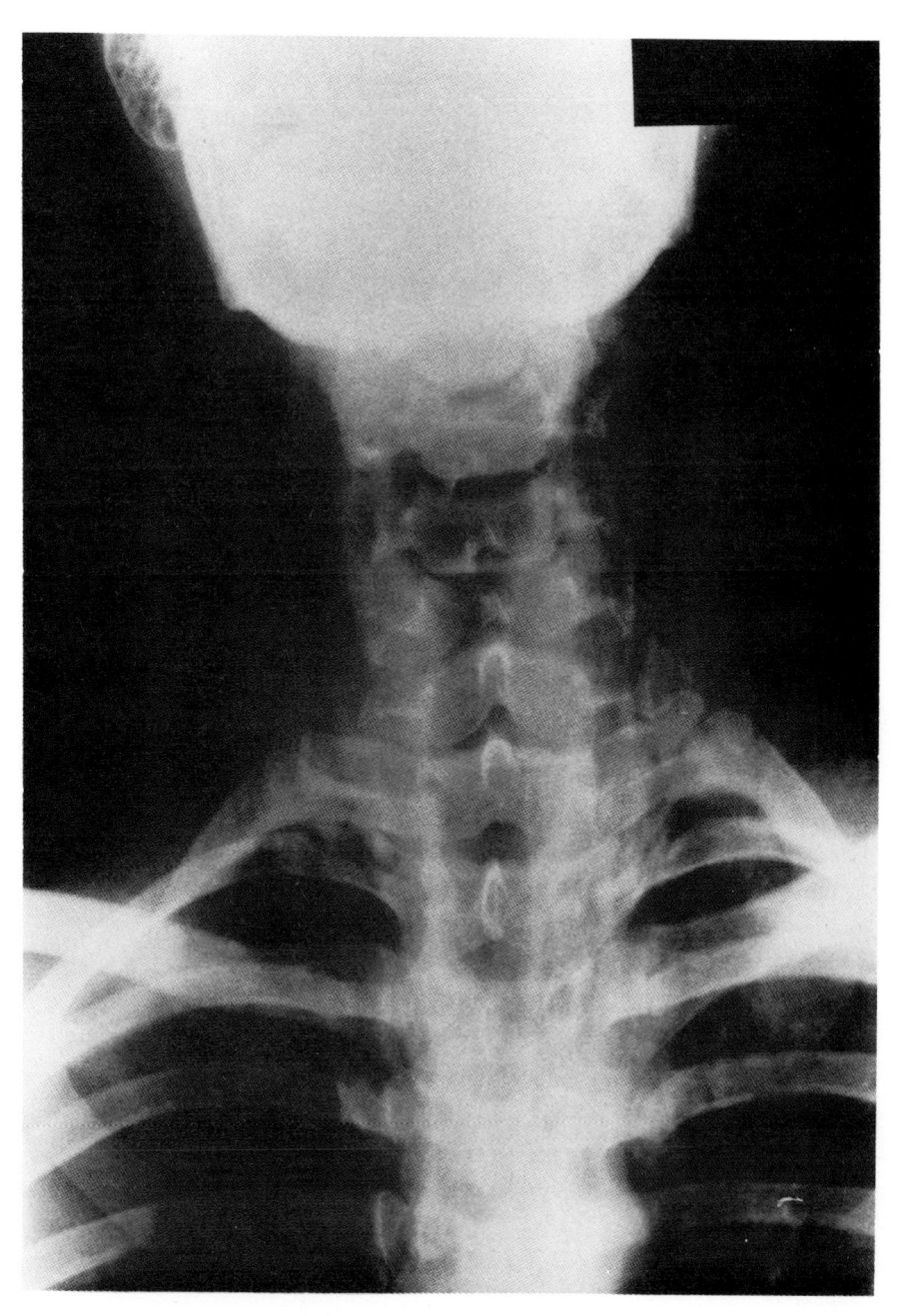

Fig 15. Case 8.

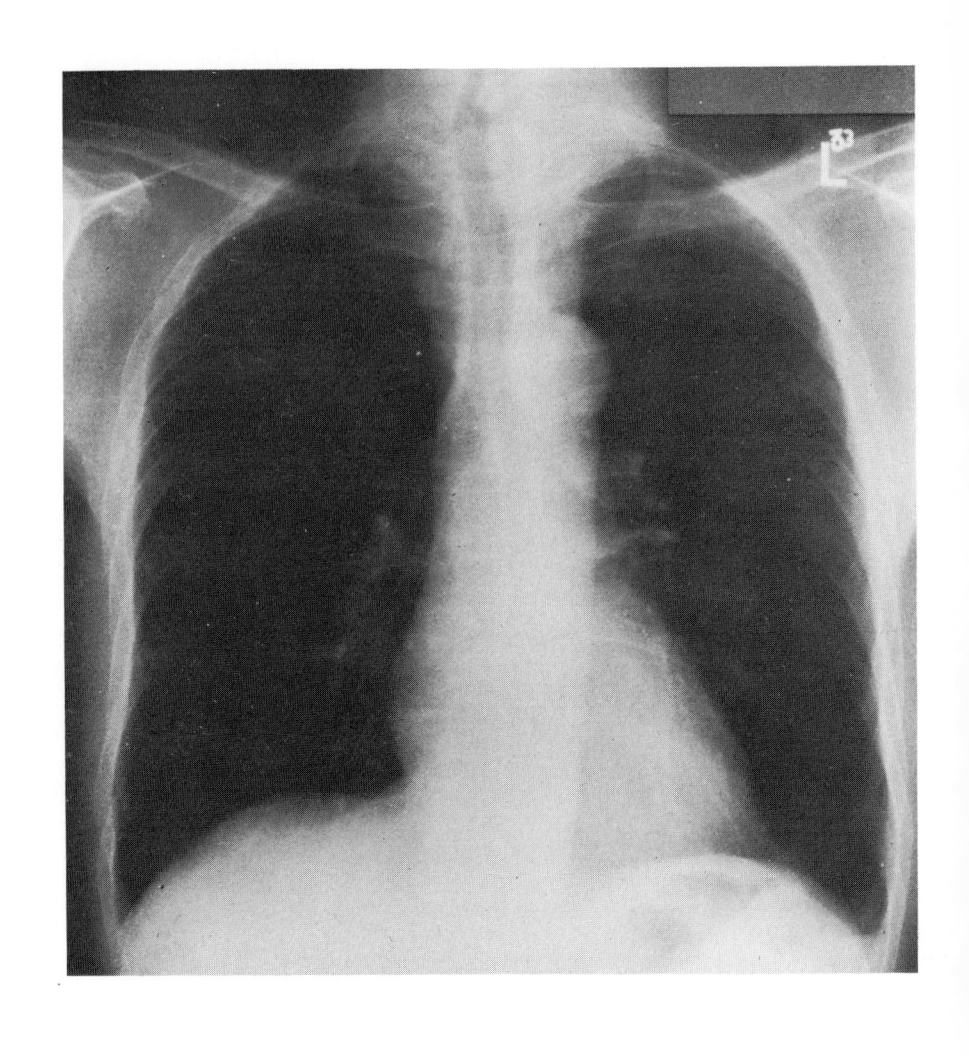

Fig 16. Case 9.

Fig 17. Case 9.

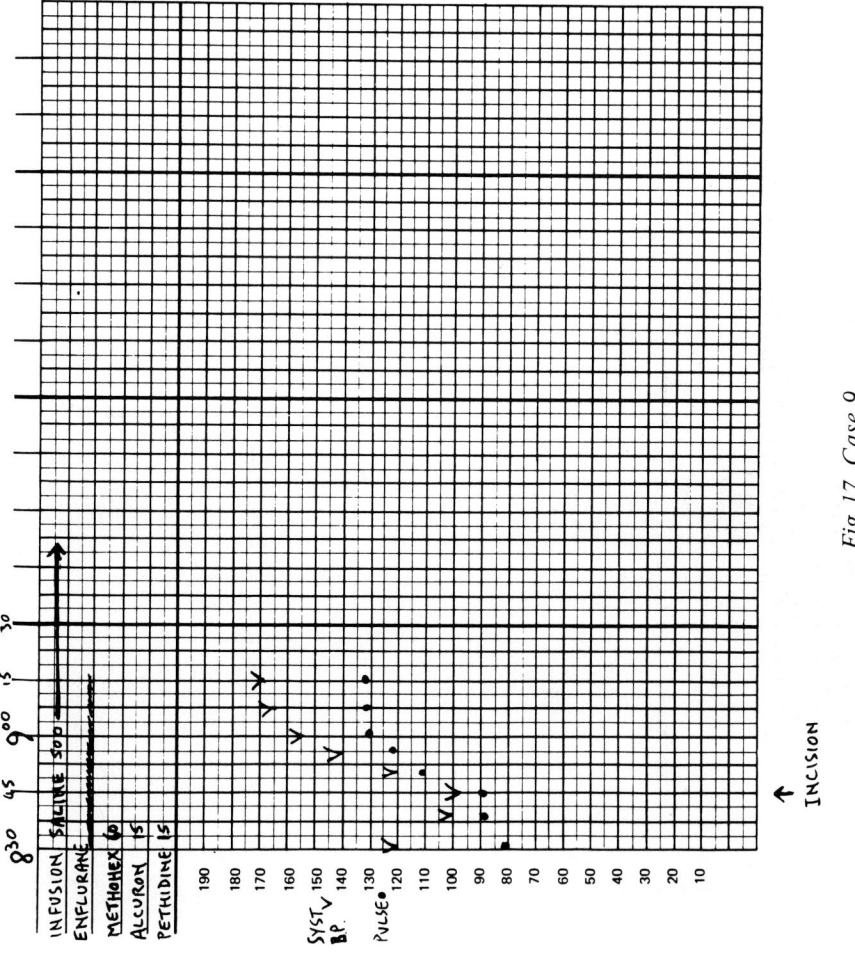

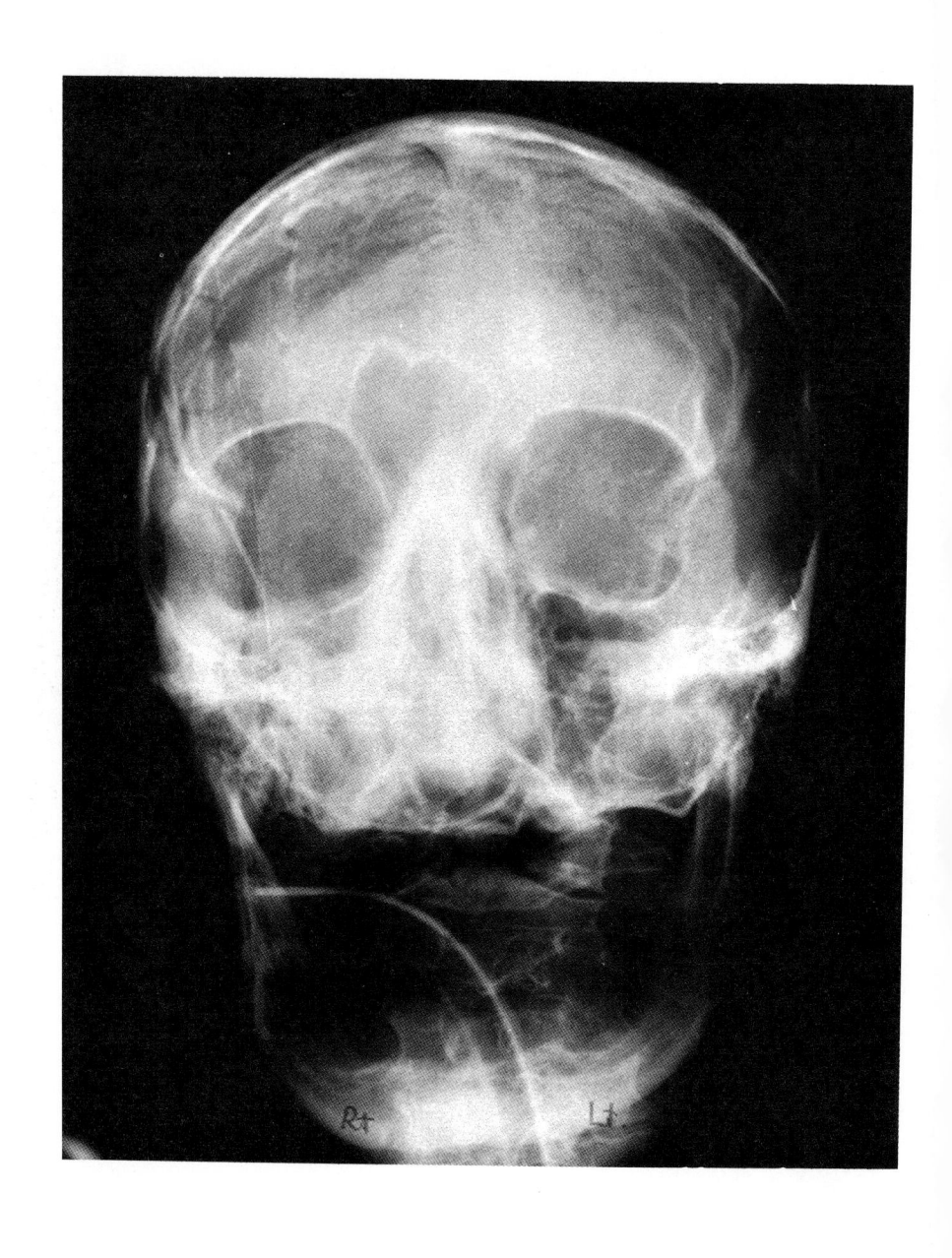

Fig 18. Case 10.

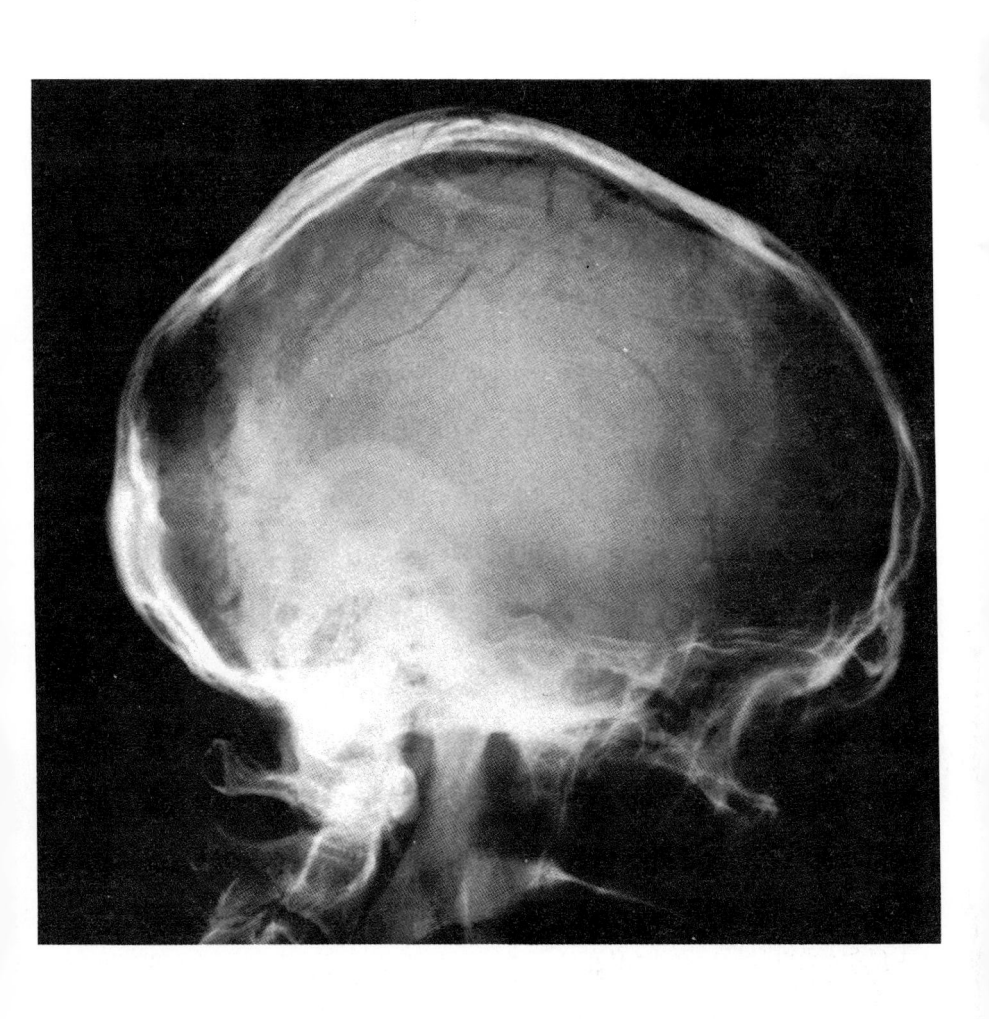

Fig 19. Case 10.

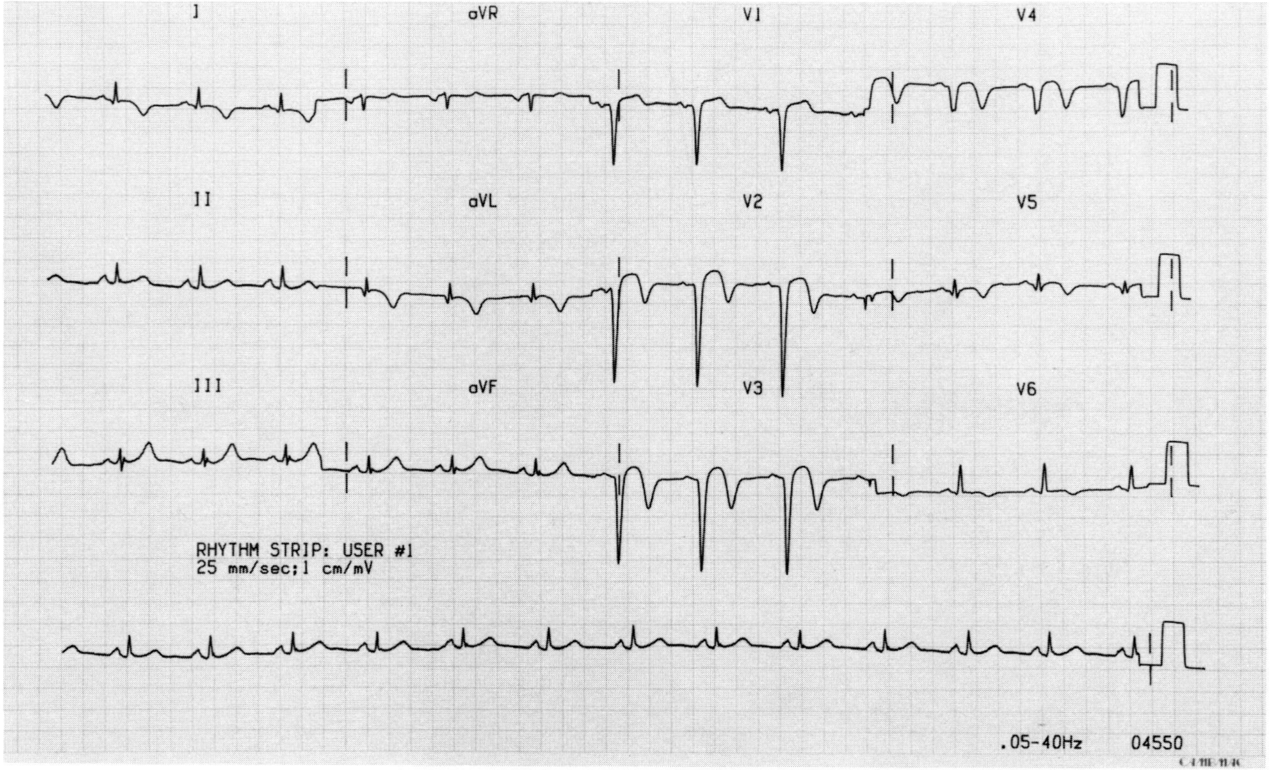

Fig 20. Case 11

Fig 21. Case 12.

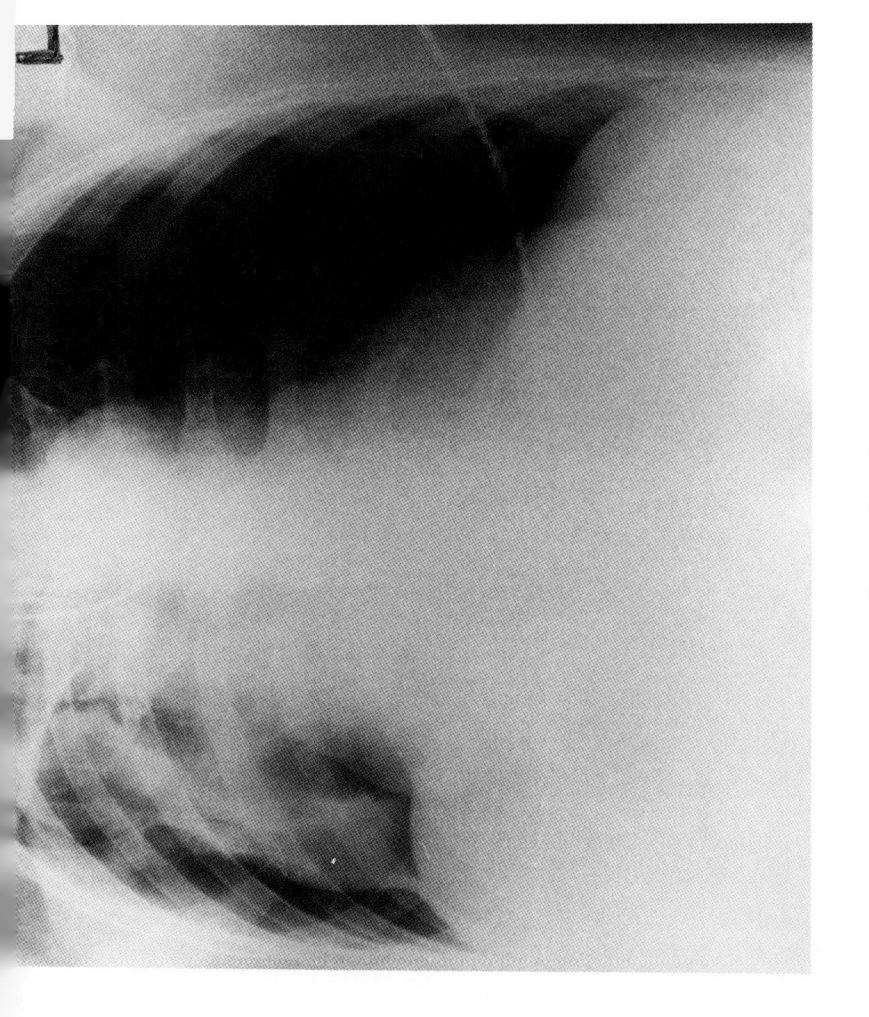

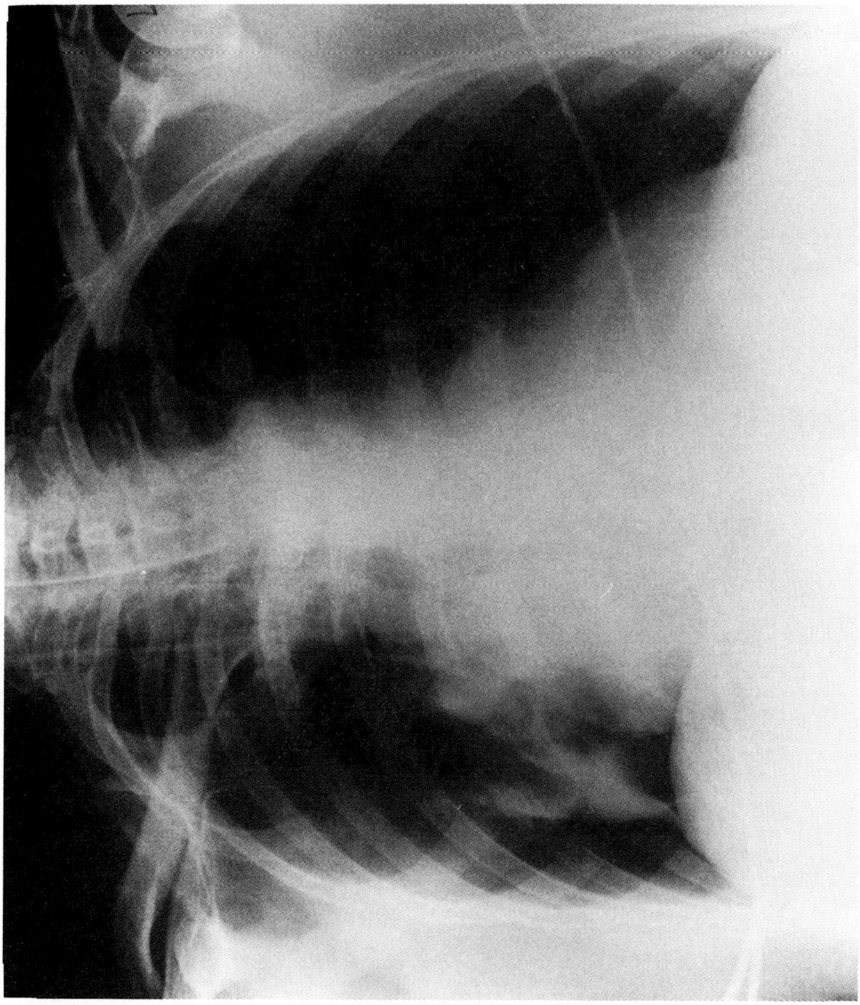

Fig 22. Case 12. 19.00 hrs.

Fig 23. Case 12. midnight.

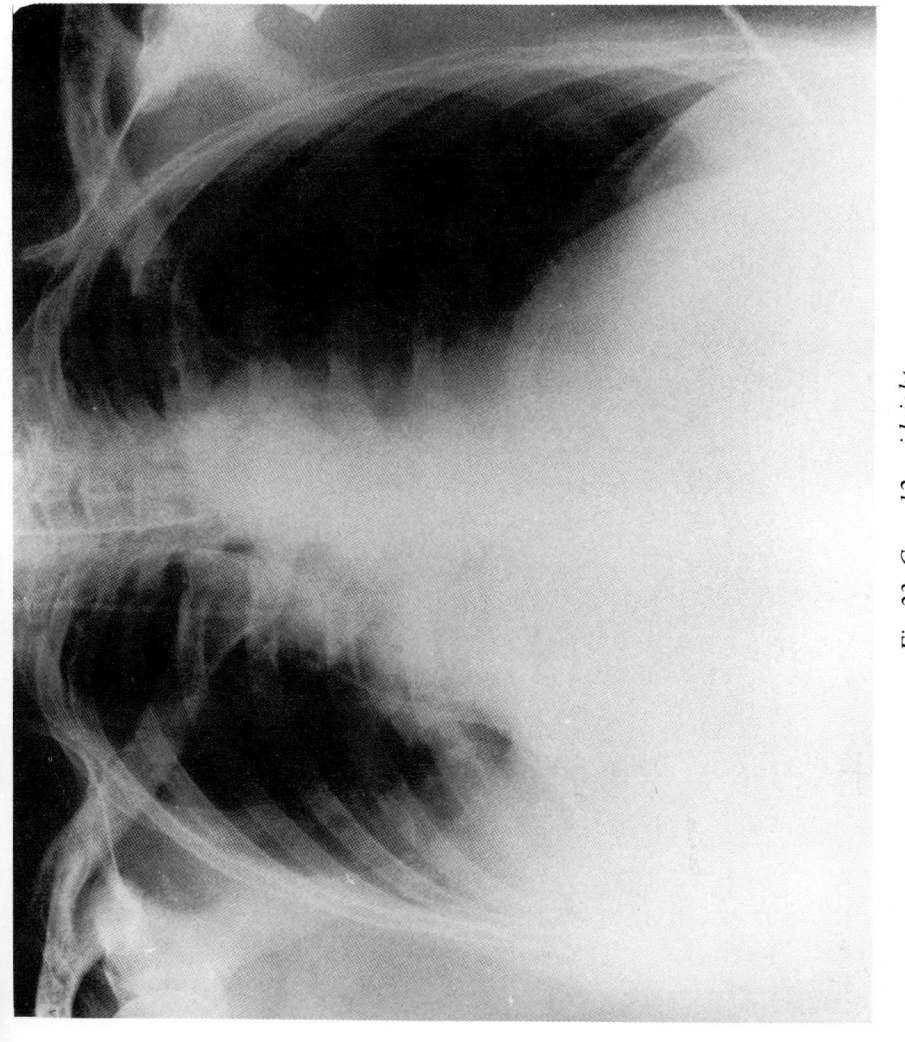

Fig 24. Case 13

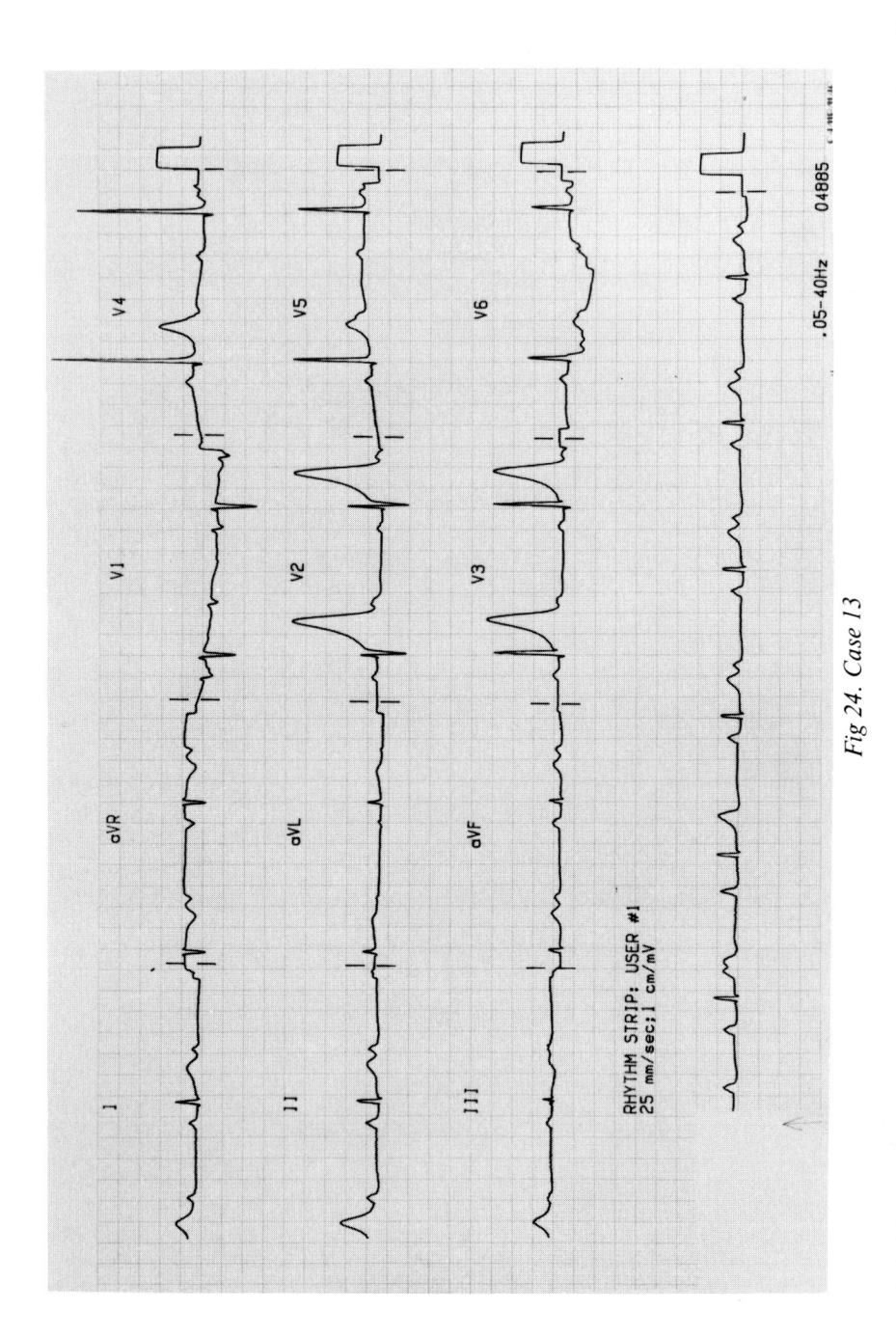

ANSWERS AND EXPLANATIONS FOR MCQ PAPERS

The correct answer options are given against each question. The abbreviations used at the end of some answers relate to the list of 'Reading and Reference Books' on page 156.

ANSWERS TO MCQ PRACTICE EXAM 1

1   A C E

Enflurane causes more respiratory depression than halothane. Both agents are depressant to the myocardium but at equal MAC enflurane is more so and causes a greater fall in cardiac output than halothane. Cardiac arrhythmias are uncommon with enflurane and there is less sensitisation of the myocardium to catecholamines than occurs with halothane, with adrenaline infiltration up to three times more may safely be given. Release of inorganic fluoride is seen with methoxyflurane and is the basis of its nephrotoxicity. More halothane is metabolised than enflurane but whereas halothane produces negligible amounts of inorganic flouride, enflurane does produce it although the levels are not high enough to cause renal problems. Boiling points - halothane 50°C, enflurane 56°C.
(S & A : p.134-137)

2   E

Intravenous regional anaesthesia was described by Bier in 1908 but he used procaine, lignocaine not being introduced until 1948. A vein on the dorsum of the hand should be chosen since if the cannula is placed proximally in a large vein with valves distally, local anaesthetic may be forced under the cuff even if it is correctly inflated to 100 mmHg above systolic pressure. Following a number of fatalities with the technique (due to various errors) bupivacaine is no longer recommended. Prilocaine 0.5% plain solution, at a dose of 3 mg/kg is the drug of choice being less likely to cause CNS toxicity than lignocaine which is also used. Sickle cell disease, both homozygous and heterozygous is an absolute contraindication to the technique because of the use of a tourniquet.
(S & A : p.332-333)

3   C D E

The approximate composition of soda lime is 90% calcium hydroxide, 5% sodium hydroxide and 1% potassium hydroxide with the addition of silicates to prevent powdering. The moisture content is 14-19% and this is essential for effective carbon dioxide absorption. Calcium carbonate is formed as the hydroxides combine with carbon dioxide in the presence of water. The size and shape of the granules is important to ensure an adequate surface area for absorption and to

MCQ Exam 1 : Answers and Explanations

minimise resistance to respiration, in a properly packed cannister half the volume should be space between the granules. Heat is produced by the chemical reaction that takes place but modern soda lime such as Durasorb, becomes much less hot than the older types. Nitrous oxide is unaffected by soda lime.
(A,R & L : p.158-159)

4   **A B**
Both halothane and enflurane relax the uterine muscle in direct proportion to the concentration used. In low dosage (halothane <0.5%) they may be used to reduce the likelihood of awareness during Caesarian section but at higher dosage they will lead to an increase in uterine bleeding, and in the case of halothane this is unresponsive to oxytocics. Neither thiopentone nor nitrous oxide affect uterine tone. In light planes of surgical anaesthesia, cyclopropane has little effect on the uterus but at deeper planes it does depress contractions. Ketamine increases uterine tone in the first and second trimesters of pregnancy but not in the third trimester.

5   **A B**
Thiopentone causes a reduction of the cardiac output by depression of myocardial contractility and peripheral vasodilatation. Severe hypotension may occur if too much is given or if the patient cannot compensate for the CVS changes, this is most likely to occur in constrictive pericarditis and tamponade, tight valvular stenosis, complete heart block, hypovolaemia and adrenocortical insufficiency. In all these conditions thiopentone must be administered with the greatest possible care. Respiratory depression with thiopentone results from depression of the respiratory centre, it depends on the dose, speed of injection and the presence of other central depressants such as opiates. Thiopentone lowers intracranial pressure, is not toxic to the liver and it is anticonvulsant.
(A,R & L : p.246-248)

6   **D**
Accurately calibrated vaporisers work on the principle that part of the flow goes through the vaporising chamber and becomes fully saturated and the rest by-passes it, the balance between the two being the 'splitting ratio'. Since SVP is 152 mmHg, fresh gas passing through the vaporiser which becomes fully saturated will have a vapour concentration of 152 divided by the atmospheric pressure, 760 mmHg and expressed as a percentage ie. 20% (as all gases are dry there is no need to consider the vapour pressure of water). Thus 80 ml of fresh gas passing through the vaporising chamber will have 20 ml of vapour added to it, making a concentration of 20%. The final

MCQ Exam 1 : Answers and Explanations

concentration is thus 20 ml in 4020 ml (the 20 ml of vapour added to the original 4 l/min of fresh gas) which is approximately 0.5%.
(H,H & T : p.78)

7 None correct
Clonidine is an antihypertensive agent, its main action is centrally stimulating α-adrenoceptors in the medulla and as these are inhibitory to the vasomotor centre the BP falls. Normal CVS reflexes are preserved and therefore problems with postural hypotension and hypotension with exercise are minimised. It will potentiate agents that lower the BP by ganglion blockade or direct action on the blood vessels and halothane should be used with care but is not contraindicated. If the BP falls excessively during anaesthesia, peripherally acting drugs such as methoxamine can be used.

Sudden withdrawal of clonidine must be avoided as metabolites of catecholamines increase markedly and this may lead to dangerous rebound hypertension.
(V,S & WS : p.339-340)

8 D
Thrombosis following an intravenous injection can follow the administration of thiopentone, etomidate and methohexitone but it is uncommon, even with etomidate and methohexitone which can cause pain on injection. Diazepam in propylene glycol is a well recognised cause of thrombophlebitis and thrombosis. Diazemuls, a formulation of diazepam as an oil/water emulsion is designed to overcome this problem and is to be preferred for the intravenous injection of diazepam.

9 A B C D E
Intravascular administration of local anaesthetic is a risk with any local block where the needle is close to blood vessels, the subclavian artery lies on the first rib immediately in front of the brachial plexus, careful aspiration prior to injection is essential. Pneumothorax is a well recognised risk and is said to have an incidence of 0.5 to 6%. If solution is injected outside the sheath of the plexus it may ascend in the tissue planes to block other nerves. The phrenic is most often involved and the diaphragm on that side will be paralysed, the risk of this and of pneumothorax leads to a general recommendation that bilateral blocks are best avoided. The vagus, recurrent laryngeal, and sympathetic nerves can also be blocked and the latter will result in Horner's syndrome.
(S & A : p.331)

MCQ Exam 1 : Answers and Explanations

10 A D E
Convulsions can occur with deep ether anaesthesia both intraoperatively and postoperatively. Hypoxia may also be the cause of convulsions particularly in the postoperative period. Local anaesthetic drugs in overdose can lead to convulsions by depression of the inhibitory centres in the brain. Neither fasciculations following suxamethonium nor the myoclonus which may be seen after halothane anaesthesia which is often incorrectly referred to as shivering, have their origin in the CNS.
(A,R & L : p.599 & 603)

11 A B C
In Mapleson's classification the Magill and the Lack circuits are type A, the latter being a coaxial version. The effort required to open the expiratory valve of the Magill circuit precludes its use in small children but it is suitable for those weighing more than 20 kg (generally over the age of 5). In spontaneously breathing patients it has been shown that the fresh gas flow can be reduced to less than the minute volume without rebreathing and hypercarbia occurring. In this situation there will be rebreathing of gas that has been in the anatomical dead space but as this has not been involved in gas exchange, it will be the same as fresh gas. Under ideal conditions the fresh gas flow can be reduced to alveolar ventilation (normally about 70% of minute volume) without rebreathing taking place and the arterial PCO_2 rising. When used for IPPV the expiratory valve must be partially closed and rebreathing will occur even at high fresh gas flows; although this may be permissible for short periods when it is not intended to lower the PCO_2, as for instance whilst waiting for the effects of suxamethonium to wear off, it is not satisfactory for longer periods of IPPV.
(S & A : p.231)

12 A E
Clinical assessment of recovery following neuromuscular block is never as reliable as the use of a nerve stimulator which should be part of the regular routine of using relaxants. In states of partial paralysis it is difficult to quantitate the degree of block with clinical signs. The ability to sustain a head lift for 5 seconds is probably the generally most useful test and it correlates well with the train of four ratio (a TOF ratio below 0.75 and most subjects cannot sustain a head lift for a full 5 seconds). Measurement of tidal volume, minute volume and end tidal CO_2 are all essentially making the same assessment and they may return to normal values even though significant residual paralysis still exists particularly in unconscious patients, they indicate only that recovery is occurring. The response to airway obstruction,

MCQ Exam 1 : Answers and Explanations

the ability to produce a negative inspiratory effort of at least -20 cm H_2O against an obstructed airway is a better indication that any residual block is not clinically significant.
(S & A : p.173)

13   B D
A haemoglobin result of under 10 g/dl is regarded as being an indication for cancelling a routine operation, although this might appear somewhat arbitrary the presence of a more marked anaemia will cause the resting cardiac output to rise so that oxygen delivery to the tissues is maintained and the patient's CVS is therefore already under increased stress. Routine urine analysis is part of the standard preoperative preparation of patients and the presence of glucose or porphyrins which may cause the urine to turn brown or red on standing, requires further investigation. The values of potassium and bilirubin given are within the normal range.

14   B C D E
At induction of anaesthesia the patient is often anxious and may have raised levels of circulating catecholamines which in the presence of volatile agents such as halothane and to a lesser extent enflurane may induce arrhythmias. Hypertensive patients are more susceptible to this problem as their hearts are already under stress. Lignocaine applied to the larynx and trachea with a spray improves the patient's tolerance of an endotracheal tube and may, if given early enough reduce the cardiovascular responses to intubation including arrhythmias. The lignocaine is rapidly absorbed and its presence in the body may also be significant. Pre-treatment with β-blockers reduces the incidence of arrhythmias, particularly those associated with intubation.

15   C E
Opinions differ as to the period for which a tourniquet can be kept inflated, indicating perhaps that a cautious approach is appropriate. The following values err towards such caution.

	Arm	Leg
Inflation time	1 hour	2 hours
Inflation pressure	systolic BP+50 mmHg	twice systolic BP

Tourniquets are associated with an increased incidence of deep vein thrombosis and should not be used in patients with HbS as acidosis and ischaemia in the limb may precipitate sickling. There is no contraindication to their use in spinal anaesthesia.
(S & A : p.451, A R & L : p.382)

MCQ Exam 1 : Answers and Explanations

16 E
It may sometimes be necessary to maintain the patient in traction for 1-2 days whilst taking measures to improve their preoperative state, but it is not reasonable to keep an elderly patient bedbound for 7-10 days prior to operation. Postoperative mortality figures of more than 25% in the over eighties are quoted, bronchopneumonia being the commonest cause of death. Early mortality has been shown to be lower and postoperative arterial hypoxaemia minimal, following local anaesthesia with spinals or epidurals but there are practical difficulties in their use. Spinal block to T10 is adequate and unilateral block, produced by keeping the patient on his side for 10-15 minutes until the local has fixed, will reduce cardiovascular changes.
(A,R & L : p.383)

17 C D
Malignant hyperpyrexia is thought to result from a defect in the control mechanism for calcium release in the sarcoplasmic reticulum and mitochondria. Dantrolene acts by reducing this calcium release and is therefore the specific agent of choice in treatment of an established case. It is given as a dose of 1 mg/kg intravenously, repeated as necessary. Mannitol is a valuable osmotic diuretic and intravenous infusion of 10-20 g may be used in malignant hyperpyrexia to maintain renal output.
(A,R & L : p.604)

18 A C D
The MAC values are cyclopropane 9.2%, enflurane 1.68%, isoflurane 1.15%, halothane 0.75%, methoxyflurane 0.16%. The value for nitrous oxide is 105% and this cannot be achieved at normal atmospheric pressure. MAC correlates with the oil/water partition coefficient and the lipid solubility of anaesthetic agents but not with the blood/gas partition coefficient.
(A,R & L : p.188)

19 A C
Cyclopropane is very explosive when mixed with oxygen over a wide range of concentrations (2.5-60%), mixed with nitrous oxide and air it is also explosive. Ether is always explosive when mixed with nitrous oxide and oxygen and in this combination is even more explosive than when mixed with oxygen alone. Halothane, enflurane, isoflurane and methoxyflurane are not explosive.
(A,R & L : p.188)

20 C E
Nodal rhythm is commonly seen with inhalational anaesthesia and is

MCQ Exam 1 : Answers and Explanations

seldom of serious significance, halothane causes a dose-dependent depression of the sinus node automaticity which will encourage the development of nodal or junctional rhythms. Fall in BP is not the cause but as with any arrhythmia, hypoxia may be the provoking factor and a careful check should be made to exclude it. Although sensory stimulation at light levels of halothane anaesthesia may lead to many types of arrhythmia, nodal rhythm is not one of them. Atropine will usually abolish a nodal rhythm but it should be administered slowly and with care as it can produce more serious ventricular arrhythmias.
(S & A : p.282-284)

21 **A**
In flutter digoxin is used as it shortens the refractory period of the myocardial cells and tends to convert the flutter to fibrillation, if the digoxin is then stopped the heart may revert to sinus rhythm. Digoxin is not of value in heart block, Stokes-Adams attacks or ventricular tachycardia. Nodal tachycardia is difficult to differentiate from other types of supraventricular tachycardia but digoxin is of no value in its treatment, and nodal tachycardia can in fact result from digoxin toxicity.
(V,S & W-S : p.370)

22 **A B C**
Dopamine has a biphasic action at lower doses it is primarily β-stimulant but at higher doses it exhibits an α-stimulant action. Infused at a rate of $10\mu g/kg/minute$ it is a β-stimulant, renal blood flow is increased by vasodilatation and stimulation of 'dopamine receptors' in the renal artery, this results in an increased urinary output and sodium output. Cardiac contractility is improved but without a rise in heart rate and the cardiac output is increased. Infused at a rate of $20\mu g/kg/minute$ or more α-stimulation predominates and multiple ventricular extrasystoles and other dysrhythmias may occur. The peripheral resistance is reduced with lower doses and increased with higher doses.
(A,R & L : p.625-626)

23 **A D**
In the CNS ketamine induces a rapid loss of consciousness and good analgesia but the unpleasant dreams and hallucinations that occur on emergence have limited its clinical use. Cerebral blood flow increases and results in an acute rise in intracranial pressure. Tone in striated muscle is slightly increased but the smooth muscle of the uterus does not relax and ketamine has been used in obstetrics. Premedication is important in reducing the hallucinations and other emergence

MCQ Exam 1 : Answers and Explanations

phenomena, benzodiazepines, droperidol and opiates have all been recommended, atropine however is not essential but may be required as in premedication for other forms of anaesthesia. It is converted to water soluble metabolites and excreted in the urine.
(A,R & L : p.269-272)

24   C E
Isoprenaline and glucagon increase the blood glucose concentration by mobilising glycogen stored in the liver. Growth hormone is diabetogenic and as well as mobilising glycogen, it inhibits the uptake of glucose into some tissues. Metformin is a biguanide and glibenclamide is a sulphonylurea, both are used in the treatment of diabetes, the former increases peripheral utilisation of glucose and the latter augments insulin secretion, they are only effective when there is some residual pancreatic β-cell activity.

25   C D E
Dantrolene is a skeletal muscle relaxant and it acts not at the neuromuscular junction but directly on the sarcoplasmic reticulum, uncoupling the excitation-contraction sequence by reducing calcium release. It is the specific agent for the treatment of malignant hyperpyrexia. Given 2 hours preoperatively it has been shown to reduce the incidence of postoperative muscle pains following the use of suxamethonium.
(A,R & L : p.305 & 605)

26   A E
As an isomer of enflurane, isoflurane has the same molecular weight. At 20°C it has a SVP of 250 mmHg, halothane is almost the same at 243 mmHg and placed in a halothane vaporiser it would give similar concentrations (there are obvious practical reasons for not doing this!). It has a MAC value of 1.15%, enflurane is 1.68%. The BP falls with isoflurane as a result of a decreased peripheral vascular resistance, changes in cardiac output are small and unlike other volatile anaesthetics, it produces minimal changes in cerebral blood flow at concentrations used for light anaesthesia.
(S & A : p.138)

27   B C
Naloxone is a specific narcotic antagonist and has no agonist activity. It antagonises the agonist actions of those analgesics which are only partial agonists, such as nalbuphine and pentazocine which may depress respiration if given in overdose. It does not however have any specific effect on respiratory depression caused by barbiturates and benzodiazepines.
(V,S & W-S : p.186-187)

MCQ Exam 1 : Answers and Explanations

28 B C D E
Thiopentone is supplied mixed with anhydrous sodium carbonate as it is only soluble in alkaline solution, the pH of a 2.5% solution being 10.5. Chemically it is the sulphur analogue of pentobarbitone, the sulphur replacing oxygen and imparting a more rapid action and recovery. In the blood about 70% is normally bound to plasma proteins and in malnutrition and other conditions where plasma proteins are low, there will be more free drug increasing the patient's sensitivity. The blood pH also effects plasma binding, raising the pH as in hyperventilation, increases the unbound portion. Thiopentone has a pKa of 7.6 and in the plasma at a pH of 7.4 about 60% is present in the non-ionised form. The clinical effects of an induction dose of thiopentone cease as the drug is redistributed in the body mainly to fat, metabolism is slow. Although traces are excreted unchanged in the urine, the majority is broken down in the liver and excreted through the kidneys and gut. About 10-15% is destroyed each hour so that at the end of 24 hours almost 30% of the original dose may remain in the body.
(A,R & L : p.245-248)

29 A C D
Hyoscine differs from atropine in its peripheral actions, by having a more potent anti-muscarinic effect on the eye and the secretions of the gut, bronchial and sweat glands; whereas atropine has a more marked action on the smooth muscle of the bronchi and GI tract as well as the heart. Both drugs are anti-emetic but hyoscine is the more effective particularly in motion sickness, hence its use for the invasion troops on D-day. It is also the better anti-sialogogue. The central action of atropine is to stimulate and then depress in high dosage, whereas hyoscine is only sedative. However there are exceptions, the anti-Parkinsonian action of atropine in reducing tremor is purely depressant and in the elderly hyoscine sometimes causes excitement and restlessness.
(V,S & W-S : p.304 & 307)

30 A B
When a nerve stimulator is used, fade and post-tetanic facilitation are characteristics of non-depolarising block blockade. Acetylcholine can itself produce a depolarising block and neostigmine by increasing its concentration at the neuromuscular junction will tend to potentiate depolarising relaxants. The presence of d-tubocurarine limits the ability of suxamethonium to get to the receptors and thereby antagonises its action. Lowering body temperature potentiates the action of depolarising agents.
(A R & L : p.285-286)

MCQ Exam 1 : Answers and Explanations

31 A B D E
Morphine and pethidine as narcotic analgesics have long been recognised to cause dependence, pentazocine although initially thought to have separated dependence from analgesia, does in fact cause psychological and physical dependence and this may be severe. Barbiturates induce emotional and physical dependence when taken over a prolonged period, stopping them leads to a withdrawal syndrome that may last up to 14 days.
(L : p.334 & 410)

32 B E
Local anaesthetics act by blocking membrane depolarisation in excitable tissues in the body, placed in proximity to peripheral nerves they block the spread of the nerve impulse and if they reach the general circulation they affect in particular the brain and conductive tissues of the heart. They are either esters (cocaine, procaine, amethocaine) or amides (lignocaine, bupivacaine, prilocaine) and are detoxified in the liver. Methaemoglobinaemia is not seen with bupivacaine but is an occasional feature of the use of prilocaine. 2 mg/kg body weight is the generally recommended maximum dose in a 4 hour period, with or without adrenaline.
(A,R & L : p.662)

33 B
For accurate measurement of the BP it is essential that the width of the cuff should be in proportion to the size of the arm. The correct width is 20% greater than the diameter of the arm and the normal adult cuff is 13 cm wide. If the cuff is too narrow in relation to the arm excessive inflation pressure will have to be generated in the cuff in order to occlude the brachial artery, and this will give an erroneously high measurement of the BP. Slow deflation of the cuff and the position of the sphygmomanometer do not affect the reading. Severe atherosclerosis may alter the pulse wave form and raise systolic pressure, but it does not alter the accuracy of the measurement.

34 None correct
The critical temperature of a gas is the temperature to which it must be cooled before it can be liquefied by pressure and the critical pressure is the pressure required to liquefy a gas at its critical temperature. For oxygen the critical temperature is -118.4°C and it can only be liquefied below this temperature. To liquefy it at -118.4°C a pressure of 50.8 atmospheres is required, this is the critical pressure. Nitrous oxide can be liquefied at room temperature as its critical temperature is 36.5°C and its critical pressure is 71.7 atmospheres.
(A,R & L : p.135)

MCQ Exam 1 : Answers and Explanations

35 B D
Poiseuille's equation states that with regard to laminar flow through tubes:

$$\text{Gas flow (Q)} = \frac{(P1-P2) \, r^4 \, \pi}{8 \, \eta \, l}$$

where (P1-P2) is the pressure drop across the tube, η the viscosity and l the length of the tube. Density is only a significant factor in turbulent flow.
(H,H & T : p.11)

36 D
Nitrogen at high pressure has a narcotic effect and this is the reason for the use of helium for diving below about 70 metres. Normal respiration is an example of laminar gas flow and viscosity is important in relation to laminar flow, but the viscosities of helium and nitrogen are similar. Helium is much less dense and in turbulent flow, as occurs in stridor and upper airway obstruction, this physical property is important; helium oxygen mixtures are therefore used in this clinical situation but this is not relevant to diving. The thermal conductivity of helium is six times greater than that of nitrogen, when helium is used in diving chambers the ambient temperature has to be kept around 30°C.

37 E
The basilic vein arises from the ulnar side of the dorsal venous arch on the back of the hand and gradually winds round the ulnar border of the forearm as it ascends to the arm, where it lies in the groove on the medial side of the biceps. Halfway up the arm it pierces the deep fascia and lies on the medial side of the brachial artery and ulnar nerve eventually becoming the axillary vein. The cephalic vein runs on the radial side of the forearm, the lateral side of the biceps and the anterior border of the deltoid to pierce the clavipectoral fascia and join the axillary vein.
(S & A : p.1-3)

38 B D
The anatomy of the first rib is of importance in relation to local blocks of the brachial plexus by the supraclavicular route and of the stellate ganglion. Moving along the upper surface of the rib from the front, the subclavian vein lies in a shallow groove anterior to the scalene tubercle into which scalenus anterior inserts. The subclavian artery crosses just behind the tubercle with the lower trunk of the brachial plexus immediately behind it, they form a deep groove. The

scalenus medius then inserts posteriorly to these structures into a roughened area on the postero-lateral area of the rib. The stellate ganglion is anterior to the head of the rib.

39 **A B D E**
The Valsalva manoeuvre is a forced expiration against a closed glottis or other obstruction and results in an increased intrathoracic pressure and a decreased venous return. Its importance to the anaesthetist is that the commencement of IPPV will lead to similar changes. The immediate response is a rise in systolic arterial pressure because the increase in intrathoracic pressure is added to the pressure of the blood in the aorta. The BP then falls as a result of a reduction in venous return, producing a drop in cardiac output. The fall in BP inhibits the baroreceptors, causing a tachycardia and a rise in peripheral resistance. When the Valsalva is released, the venous return and cardiac output are restored but the peripheral vessels are still constricted. The BP now rises above normal, the baroreceptors are stimulated and a bradycardia occurs until the BP returns to normal.
(G : p.485)

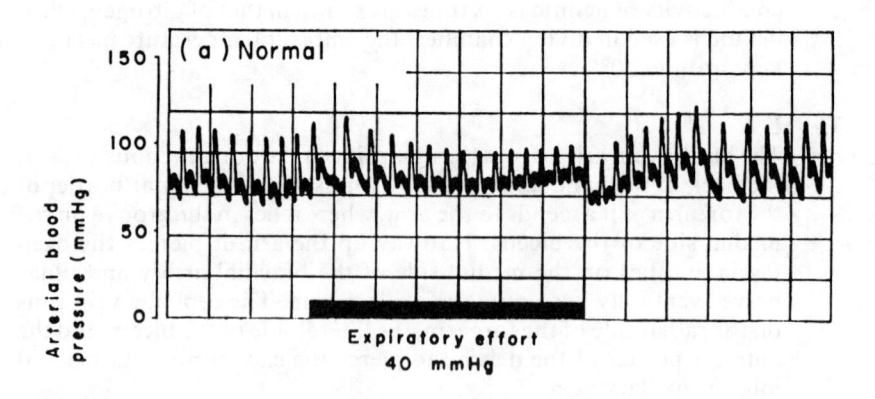

Normal Valsalva

40 **A D E**
The molecular weight of albumin is approximately 65,000 and the normal blood level is 34-45 g/l. Although it has a lower molecular weight than globulin it makes a significant contribution to the plasma oncotic pressure because there is considerably more of it. Malabsorption syndrome and liver disease result in a fall in albumin.
(G : p.429-430)

MCQ Exam 1 : Answers and Explanations

41 A E
In sleep there is central depression of respiration. A rise in body temperature will increase metabolism and CO_2 production so increasing ventilation. Acidaemia will stimulate respiration to reduce arterial PCO_2 leading to a compensatory respiratory alkalosis. In hypothermia the respiration is reduced, whereas at altitude it is increased due to the hypoxic drive induced by the low PO_2.

42 A B E
The oxygen dissociation curve is moved to the right by:
Rise in hydrogen ions : acidosis, pH decrease
Rise in body temperature
Rise in PCO_2 : in the pulmonary capillaries PCO_2 falls
Rise in 2,3-DPG : in anaemia this is raised
The arterial PO_2 falls with increasing age but this does not affect the dissociation curve.
(H,H & T : p.127-128)

43 C E
The knee jerk response is a stretch reflex and can be elicited by tapping the patella tendon, which stimulates the muscle spindle 1A afferents. The reflex is monosynaptic, not involving any interneurones. The sensory impulse synapses with the anterior horn cells at L 3-4 and it is not controlled by the higher centres although it may be modified by them. Although Golgi tendon organs are present in the patella tendon, they play no part in the knee jerk.
(H,H & T : p.175)

44 A C D E
Carbon dioxide is transported in a variety of ways in the blood:
1. Dissolved in simple solution in both the plasma and red cells.
2. Most of the CO_2 is hydrolysed to carbonic acid in the red cells but this then dissociates to hydrogen ions and bicarbonate. Bicarbonate then diffuses into the plasma in exchange for chloride ions, the chloride shift.
3. As carbamino compounds in combination with haemoglobin and to lesser extent with plasma proteins.
(G : p.538-539)

45 A B C D E
Acute adaptation to the hypoxia of high altitude involves an increase in respiratory minute volume mediated by the peripheral chemoreceptors which are sensitive to hypoxia; the increased respiration leads to a reduction in the arterial CO_2 level. Initially this hyperventilation is reversible if oxygen is administered but after about a week it becomes irreversible. There is tachycardia and an increase in cardiac output but the CVS changes are much smaller than the respiratory.

There is an increase in 2,3-DPG levels stimulated by hypoxia and this leads to a decreased affinity of haemoglobin for oxygen making more oxygen available in the tissues and shifting the oxygen dissociation curve to the right despite the fact that respiratory alkalosis would be tending to move the curve to the left. Polycythaemia develops over some months and increases oxygen carrying capacity.
(G : p.553-554)

46 A D
The normal PR interval is from 0.12 to 0.2 seconds and it represents the period between atrial depolarisation and conduction through the AV node. The resting membrane potential of the myocardial fibres is -80 millivolts and the T wave represents ventricular repolarisation. Although the S wave represents the end of the electrical stimulation of the ventricles the mechanical changes lag well behind, the S wave occurs during early systole.
(G : p.436-439)

47 A C D E
The glomerular filtration rate (GFR) is maintained at a steady level over a wide range of arterial BP as a result of autoregulation in the kidney. The pH of the urine varies widely from extremes of 4.5 to about 8.0, renal compensation for changes in the blood pH are slow and in hypokalaemia the need to retain potassium leads to the loss of hydrogen ions even though a metabolic alkalosis is present in the blood, thus renal pH does not always reflect blood pH. Both urinary sodium and osmolality can vary widely but the levels given in the question are normal values. Creatinine clearance is a convenient way of assessing GFR.

48 A B C
The 'a', 'c' and 'v' waves seen in the central venous pulse are produced by pressure changes in the right atrium which are transmitted to the great veins. The 'a' wave is caused by atrial systole which results in the regurgitation of some blood back into the great veins, it is absent in atrial fibrillation. The 'c' wave is caused by bulging of the tricuspid valve into the atrium during the phase of isometric ventricular contraction and the 'v' wave results from the pressure rise as blood flows into the RA but when the tricuspid valve opens and blood can enter the RV the pressure falls.

In inspiration, expansion of the chest creates a negative pressure which is transmitted to the veins in the chest and the central venous pressure falls. Clinically there is often a difference in the performance of the left and right sides of the heart. To obtain meaningful information when the problem is related to the left side, a balloon-tipped catheter can be used to measure the pulmonary capillary wedge pressure which is closely related to the left atrial pressure. (G : p.454)

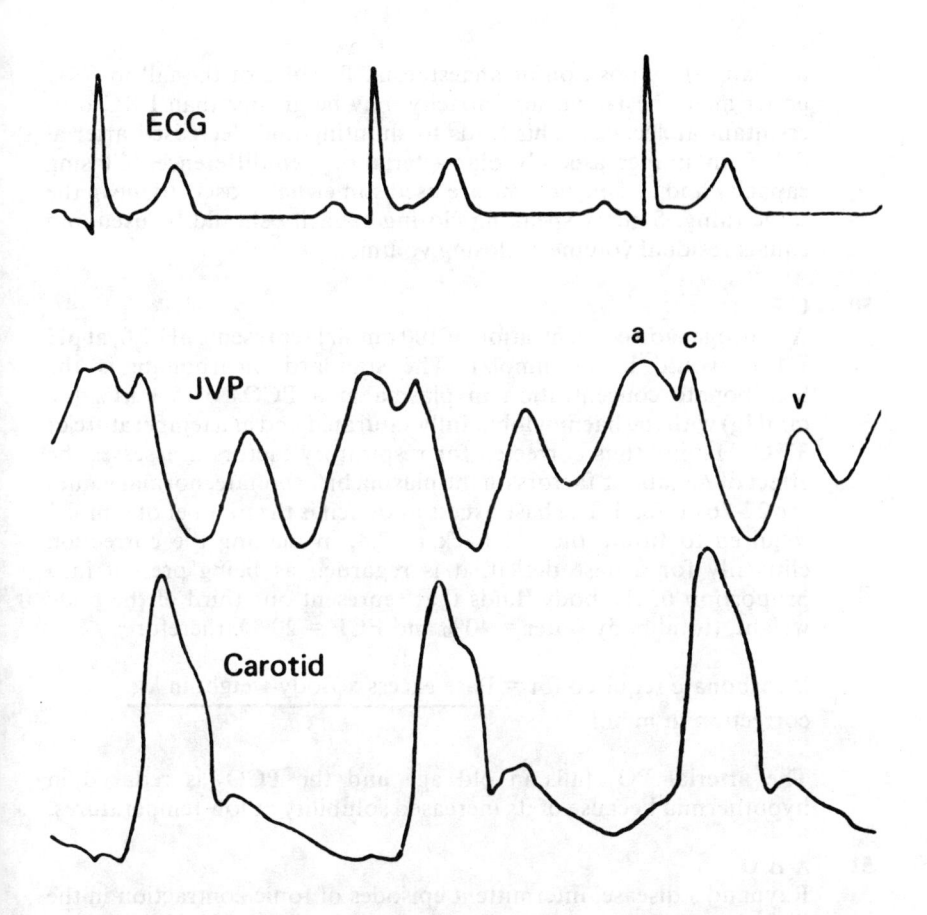

49 **B E**
The functional residual capacity (FRC) is the volume in the lungs at the end of expiration and represents the resting position of the lungs. There is probably a slight increase in FRC with age. Much more significant is the fall in FRC that occurs on moving from the upright to the supine position, and the further fall in FRC that occurs when a supine patient is anaesthetised. This fall on induction is of the order of 20% and is similar whether there is spontaneous breathing or IPPV. Closing capacity is the lung volume at which airways start to close. In contrast to FRC it does increase markedly with age, but is

MCQ Exam 1 : Answers and Explanations

unchanged by position or anaesthesia. Because of the fall in FRC under anaesthesia, closing capacity may be greater than FRC with resultant atelectasis. This leads to shunting and decreased arterial PO_2 with an increased alveolar-arterial oxygen difference. (Closing capacity and closing volume are used somewhat loosely to mean the same thing. Strictly speaking closing capacity should be used and equals residual volume + closing volume).

50 C E
A hydrogen ion concentration of 100 nmol/l represents pH 7.0, at pH 7.4 it would be 40 nmol/l. The standard bicarbonate is the bicarbonate concentration in plasma at a PCO_2 of 5.3 kPa (40 mmHg) with the haemoglobin fully saturated and at a temperature of 37°C. Having thus corrected for respiratory factors it assesses the effect of metabolic factors on the plasma bicarbonate, normal values are 22-26 mmol/l. The base excess or deficit is the number of mmol/l required to titrate the pH back to 7.4, in making the correction clinically for a base deficit, it is regarded as being present in a proportion of the body fluids that represent one third of the body weight, (total body water = 40% and ECF = 20%), therefore:

Bicarbonate required for = Base excess x Body weight in kg
correction in mmol   3

The arterial PO_2 falls in old age and the PCO_2 is reduced in hypothermia because of its increased solubility at low temperatures.

51 A B D
Raynaud's disease, intermittent episodes of tonic contraction in the digital arteries, may occur in the primary idiopathic form as an exaggerated response to cold more common in young women or as the secondary type, Raynaud's phenomenon, resulting from a variety of causes such as arteriosclerosis, cervical rib, the use of vibrating tools and cryoglobinaemia. Although more common in the hands, it does occur in the feet; ischaemic changes and even gangrene may develop. The response to treatment with vasodilators or sympathectomy is very often disappointing.
(D : p.199)

52 A C
Chronic deficiency of hormones of the adrenal cortex is Addison's disease and is associated with the loss of sodium from the body leading to a low serum sodium and low BP. The serum potassium rises and the skin pigmentation increases. Abdominal striae are seen

MCQ Exam 1 : Answers and Explanations

in Cushing's syndrome which is due to an excessive secretion of hormones from the adrenal cortex.
(D : p.447-448)

53 A B
Chronic bronchitis develops in response to the long continued action of various types of irritant, particularly cigarette smoke, on the bronchial mucosa. It is characterised by increased mucus secretion and mucosal oedema which tend to block the bronchioles and result in alveolar air trapping in expiration. This alveolar distension leads to an increase in residual volume. The FEV_1/FVC ratio falls and in severe cases may be as low as 30% (normal 70%). Although some patients die within a few years, others survive for many years with a gradually diminishing respiratory reserve.
(D : p.252-253)

54 A B C D E
Angina pectoris, pain due to myocardial ischaemia, can result from any situation in which the coronary blood flow and the supply of oxygen is insufficient for the needs of the myocardium. Although coronary atheroma is the commonest cause, polyarteritis can also constrict the coronary vessels. Anaemia reduces the supply of oxygen to the coronary circulation and increases the cardiac output in order to satisfy the oxygen requirements of the tissues. Aortic stenosis and paroxysmal ventricular tachycardia both increase the work of the myocardium and may lead to angina. Angina pectoris is a recognised feature of myxoedema and results from the widespread degenerative vascular disease and hypertension which are often present in this condition.
(D : p.167 & 436)

55 A E
The absorption into the circulation of irrigating fluids used at TURP's is well recognised. There is dilutional hyponatraemia which can cause confusion, convulsions and coma, pulmonary oedema, acute left heart failure and cardiac arrest. Glycine 1.5% is isotonic which prevents haemolysis.
(A,R & L : p.363-364)

56 D
P waves on the ECG are the result of the electrical activity of synchronous atrial contraction, they will be present in complete heart block where the atria contract normally but the impulse fails to be conducted to the ventricles and P waves occur independently of QRS complexes. In ventricular tachycardia, ventricular contraction origi-

nates from an abnormal focus in the ventricles and only abnormal QRS complexes are seen. Supraventricular tachycardia results from either re-entry of electrical activity or rapidly firing abnormal foci in the atria and P waves are not usually seen. In flutter atrial contraction is asynchronous, whereas in nodal rhythm the electrical impulse starts in the AV node and progresses both forwards into the ventricles and backwards into the atria, the result is that that P wave is either lost in the QRS complex or appears after it, inverted.

57 A C
A rise in serum potassium is characteristic of the onset of renal failure but changes in the serum sodium are more variable being dependent on a variety of factors but a fall to 125 mmol may occur. Adrenocortical insufficiency, with reduced cortisol and aldosterone secretion can also produce these changes.

Hypopituitarism results from destruction of the anterior lobe of the pituitary but although symptoms of adrenal insufficiency and low BP may develop, aldosterone is still produced and electrolyte changes are not seen. Cushing's syndrome in which cortisol is raised and primary aldosteronism (Conn's syndrome) in which aldosterone is raised, would tend to result in the opposite electrolyte changes.
(V : p.143 & 465-478, D : p.700)

58 A C D E
In carcinoma of the gallbladder, gallstones are usually present but the part they play in its aetiology is unclear. Obstruction of the bile duct can lead to infection and ascending cholangitis which may result in liver abscesses or septicaemia. If the obstruction is lower down then pancreatitis may also be present. Rarely gallstones reach the intestinal tract, usually via a cholecystenteric fistula and can then cause intestinal obstruction.
(D : p.371 & 374)

59 B D
Emphysema and chronic bronchitis represent two extremes of a clinical spectrum and many patients have features of both. However there are patients who fall into one of the two traditional categories of pink puffer or blue bloater. Pink puffers are typically dyspnoeic with hyperinflation but usually maintain a normal arterial PCO_2 and a reasonable PO_2. In contrast blue bloaters have a raised arterial PCO_2 and a lower PO_2 probably as a result of reduced sensitivity of the respiratory centre to CO_2 as well as the increased work of breathing. As a result of chronic respiratory acidosis they develop a compensatory metabolic alkalosis with a raised standard bicar-

bonate. They also have polycythaemia because of chronic hypoxaemia. Transfer factor is lower in the emphysematous patient because of the loss of alveolar walls resulting in less area for the diffusion of carbon monoxide.

60 C
In sickle cell trait both normal adult haemoglobin, HbA, and between 25% and 45% of abnormal HbS are present in the blood, the condition is therefore designated HbAS. A Sickledex test screens for HbS and is positive in both homozygous and heterozygous individuals, only electrophoresis can differentiate between the two. Red cell survival is normal and anaemia is not usually present in uncomplicated HbAS, nor is splenomegaly. Unexplained haematuria is seen and there is also a reduced ability to concentrate urine. For patients with sickle cell trait a carefully conducted anaesthetic with continuous attention to adequate oxygen supply is all that is required, measures such as exchange transfusion need only be considered for full sickle cell disease.
(V : p.349-350)

ANSWERS TO MCQ PRACTICE EXAM 2

The correct answer options are given against each question number.

1 B D E
Halothane is not inflammable and may safely be used with soda lime in closed circuit anaesthesia. It causes dilatation in the cerebral circulation leading to a rise in ICP and when the ICP is already raised as in head injuries, it should be used with caution if at all. In the presence of halothane anaesthesia the threshold for dysrhythmias with catecholamines is lowered, if exogenous catecholamines are used as with adrenaline infiltration by the surgeon, this must be taken into account. Although opinions differ, a general recommendation is that not more than 10 ml of adrenaline solution at a maximum concentration of 1 in 100,000 should be used in a 10 minute period or 30 ml in 1 hour, the ventilation being normal. The reduction of uterine tone makes halothane an unsuitable agent at normal concentrations for Caesarian section and ERCP.
(A,R & L : p.198 : 200)

2 C E
An endotracheal tube that is too long is more likely to pass into the right main bronchus than the left as the latter branches at a more acute angle. Occlusion of the secondary bronchus to the right upper

MCQ Exam 2 : Answers and Explanations

lobe which branches off to the right 2.5 cm below the carina, will eventually cause collapse of the right upper lobe but not within 5 minutes. Collapse of the left lung increases intrapulmonary shunting and results in a reduction of the uptake of less soluble gases such as oxygen leading to hypoxaemia but not hypotension. Likewise the uptake of relatively insoluble anaesthetic gases or volatile agents will be reduced. By comparison, maintaining the ventilation allows a soluble gas such as CO_2 to be effectively eliminated.

3   **A B E**
Malignant hyperpyrexia, a condition in which uncontrolled muscle activity leads to excessive heat production and a rise in body temperature exceeding 2°C per hour, can be triggered by a variety of drugs of which halothane and suxamethonium are the most frequently implicated. Although onset is usually during anaesthesia, late onset in the recovery is described. Muscle rigidity is often noted following suxamethonium administration but tubocurarine has no effect on this as it arises in the muscle itself and not the neuromuscular junction. The CPK rises to very high levels although this alone is not diagnostic, neither is simple muscle histology. A muscle biopsy is needed for in vitro exposure testing if the diagnosis is to be confirmed.

4   **A B E**
Depolarising muscle relaxants such as suxamethonium and decamethonium cause depolarisation of the motor end-plate of the same kind as that produced by acetylcholine, but the block persists. Excessive dosage with neostigmine and edrophonium can lead to such a build up of acetylcholine, due to inhibition of cholinesterase that a depolarising block results. It is therefore recommended that not more than 5 mg of neostigmine be given to reverse non-depolarising muscle relaxants. Gallamine and atracurium are non-depolarising muscle relaxants.
(A,R & L : p.283 & 295)

5   **A C E**
Chemically ethers have an oxygen molecule in their carbon chain, methoxyflurane, enflurane and isoflurane are all halogenated ethers, the latter two being isomers. Halothane is a halogenated hydrocarbon and cyclopropane a hydrocarbon but with no halogen atoms.

6   **D E**
Trichlorethylene has a SVP of 60 mmHg at 20°C and therefore has a low volatility. Although it has an obvious smell, it is not regarded as being very irritant to the respiratory tract but tachypnoea is a

MCQ Exam 2 : Answers and Explanations

common feature of its use. It has been shown to produce no significant alteration in forearm blood flow and is not a vasodilator. With soda lime and the presence of heat trichlorethylene can be broken down to produce toxic substances, chiefly dichloracetylene which can cause paralysis of cranial nerves. Modern soda lime is much less likely to get sufficiently hot for this reaction to take place. (A,R & L : p.194-198)

7 **D**
MCQ questions involving clinical situations require a cautious approach as in reality such situations are rarely clearly defined. First analyse the data provided, the PCO_2 is raised and the cardiovascular changes described could be secondary to this. There is arterial hypoxaemia. A simple serum bicarbonate will be influenced by the PCO_2 unlike a standard bicarbonate value, but a result at the upper end of the normal range rules out a metabolic acidosis. Septicaemia is characterised by a fall in BP. Transfusion initially will lead to a rise in the CVP and cardiovascular parameters may improve, but overtransfusion overloads the right and left sides of the heart and the BP falls. Segmental pulmonary collapse results in increased intrapulmonary shunting and arterial hypoxaemia, but if ventilation is maintained in the rest of the lung, CO_2 elimination is unchanged and the arterial PCO_2 does not rise. The changes described can occur with underventilation in the post-operative period resulting in hypercarbia and hypoxaemia.

8 **A B C**
In overdose local anaesthetic drugs are depressant to the CVS and CNS. Hypotension and cardiovascular collapse may occur but in the CNS stimulation precedes depression, probably as a result of inhibitory centres being blocked first. Restlessness with involuntary movements and convulsions may be seen before loss of consciousness and respiratory depression.

9 **B D E**
Warming blood reduces the incidence of arrhythmias due to hypothermia, acidosis and hyperkalaemia. Blood should not be left out of the refrigerator for long periods to rewarm as this does increase the risk of infection but the use of standard blood warmers is satisfactory. Increasing the temperature of blood shifts the oxygen dissociation curve to the right. Gases are more soluble in liquids at lower temperatures (cold lager is less fizzy), so that in blood as the temperature rises less is dissolved and the partial pressure rises, this is more marked with a soluble gas such as CO_2 than with a less soluble one, such as O_2. Thus for CO_2:

PCO_2 at 20°C = 15 mmHg
PCO_2 at 37°C = 34.8 mmHg
(A,R & L : p.883 & 348)

10 A B
Etomidate commonly causes pain at the site of injection particularly if the injection is made into a small vein; although it is water soluble the commercially available preparation is made up with 35% propylene glycol which reduces, but does not abolish the incidence of pain. Methohexitone also commonly causes pain on injection but paradoxically is less likely than thiopentone which does not cause pain, to lead to tissue damage if injected subcutaneously or intra-arterially; this is probably due to the use of a lower concentration of methohexitone.

11 A B E
In the obese the functional residual capacity falls and the closing capacity encroaches into it so as to lie within the range of the tidal volume, this leads to increased ventilation-perfusion mismatch and arterial hypoxaemia. The Pickwickian syndrome in which airway problems, particularly during sleep, lead to hypoventilation and hypercarbia can also occur but is less common than hypoxaemia. Intubation is often technically difficult, a laryngoscope with a long blade and a stilette for the endotracheal tube should be available. Although the assessment of drug dosage in the obese may be more difficult, in relating their lean body mass and fat to the drug being used, there is no specific increase in sensitivity in these patients to either thiopentone or the non-depolarising muscle relaxants.
(S & A : p.481)

12 D
There is no standard 'cockpit drill' for checking anaesthetic machines prior to use but the small booklet issued by BOC Medishield Service Division can be recommended. To ensure that the correct gases are connected to the correct flowmeter tests such as 'the single hose test', require disconnection of the anaesthetic machine from the pipeline supply and the reinsertion of the oxygen pipe and then the nitrous oxide pipe in turn whilst checking the oxygen flowmeter to ensure that it alone is influenced by oxygen flow. Modern oxygen alarms sound an audible warning activated by falling oxygen pressure alone, but the diversion of the nitrous oxide supply through the whistle prolongs this audible warning. When checking for leaks it is recommended that vaporisers be turned off.

A pressure relief valve set at 30 kPa is fitted on the Boyles machine,

MCQ Exam 2 : Answers and Explanations

this is intended to protect the machine not the patient and should open when the gas outlet is occluded. Interlocks were at one time fitted to anaesthetic machines to prevent the use of trichlorethylene with the closed circuit, but the confusion caused by the possibility of their being inadvertently turned on led to their being discontinued. (A R & L : p.147, 151)

13 A B D E
Antigenic reactions are more frequent with larger molecular weight Dextrans and Dextran 110 is no longer available for this reason. Dextran 70 produces reactions in about 0.2% of cases, this is usually only a mild pyrexia but in patients with a history of asthma or allergy it may be more severe and circulatory collapse has been described. Infusion of more than 1.5 litres in a 24 hour period may lead to problems with cross-matching tests as a result of rouleaux formation, this is more likely to occur with high molecular weight Dextrans. As they decrease blood viscosity and thereby increase blood flow, Dextrans are used in prophylaxis against DVT's. In dehydrated patients, Dextran 40 may produce a viscous glomerular filtrate which causes renal tubular obstruction leading to renal failure.

14 A D
In healthy individuals suxamethonium administration results in a rise in serum potassium of about 0.2-0.4 mmol/l and although pre-treatment with a small dose of d-tubocurarine may limit this rise, by itself d-tubocurarine has no effect on the serum potassium. Thiopentone produces a small decrease. In patients with extensive tissue breakdown such as trauma and burns (particularly between 3 and 10 weeks) the serum potassium is raised and suxamethonium may be particularly dangerous. In metabolic acidosis hydrogen ions enter cells in exchange for potassium ions thus raising plasma potassium. In alkalosis there is increased entry of potassium ions into cells as well as increased loss of potassium in the urine as hydrogen ions are retained, the plasma potassium therefore falls.

15 A B C D E
Fat embolism is often associated with fractures of the femur and tibia and its onset may be soon after the injury or delayed 2-3 days, it may be wrongly diagnosed as shock. The deposition of fat droplets in the lungs can lead to major respiratory problems, dyspnoea, pallor, cyanosis and pyrexia occur, the arterial PO_2 will fall and respiratory distress can develop. Fat may be found in the sputum and urine and the appearance of petechial haemorrhages over the upper chest, neck and in the conjunctiva is a characteristic sign, usually seen on the second or third day. Fat in the cerebral circulation and hypoxaemia

can lead to mental deterioration and coma as well as being an additional cause of pyrexia.
(A,R & L : p.848-849)

16   A E
Non-depolarising or competitive muscle relaxants are characterised by fade and post-tetanic facilitation when tested with a nerve stimulator. The response of non-depolarising muscle relaxants to acidosis and alkalosis is not uniform but d-tubocurarine and pancuronium both have their action prolonged by acidosis and shortened by alkalosis, depolarising muscle relaxants are affected in the opposite way. Severe hypothermia (below 30°C) increases the block with non-depolarising muscle relaxants. Fasciculation and dual block are features of depolarising muscle blockade.
(A,R & L : p.285-286)

17   B C D
Medical oxygen is manufactured by the fractional distillation of liquid air, it has a critical temperature of -118.4°C (nitrous oxide is 36.5°C). With oil and grease at high pressure ignition can occur and these substances must never be applied to seal leaks at the cylinder yoke. Hyperbaric oxygen, usually at 2-2.5 atmospheres can be used for a variety of medical conditions, but acute oxygen toxicity and convulsions are recognised complications of its use. Bone marrow depression can occur with the prolonged use of nitrous oxide.
(A,R & L : p.218 & 816)

18   A B C
Arthur E. Guedel (1883-1956) an American anaesthetist described his signs of anaesthesia in relation to the administration of open ether and spontaneous respiration, but they have a general application for all inhalational anaesthetics. Briefly they consist of:

First stage	Analgesia
Second stage	Excitement
Third stage	Surgical anaesthesia
Plane 1	Onset of automatic respiration to cessation of eyeball movement
Plane 2	Cessation of eyeball movement to start of intercostal paralysis
Plane 3	Start to completion of intercostal paralysis
Plane 4	Completion of intercostal paralysis to diaphragmatic paralysis
Fourth stage	Overdosage

MCQ Exam 2 : Answers and Explanations

The respiration is irregular in stage 2 and becomes regular and automatic at the start of stage 3. The pupils are usually dilated in the first stage due to emotion, in the second stage dilatation is the result of sympathetic stimulation of the dilator pupillae. In the third stage, plane 1, they return to normal and then progressively dilate again until the fourth stage. Premedication with opiates and atropine will affect these responses, miosis produced by the opiate usually predominates.
(A,R & L : p.168-169)

19 B C E
Nitrous oxide is produced by heating ammonium nitrate above 240°C in an iron retort. Ammonia, nitric acid, nitrogen, nitric oxide (NO) and nitrogen dioxide (NO_2) are also produced. The ammonia and nitric acid are reconstituted to ammonium nitrate and removed. The remaining gases pass through a series of scrubbers in which they are washed with water and caustic soda to remove all the NO and NO_2 this is carefully monitored but contamination of nitrous oxide has occurred and both contaminants are toxic. A crude test for contamination is to place a piece of moistened starch-iodide paper into a large syringe and draw in the suspect nitrous oxide along with 25% oxygen, if the gas is contaminated the paper turns blue within 10 minutes.

Full cylinders contain up to 80% of liquid nitrous oxide. In continuous use there is some fall in the gauge pressure this results from the drop in temperature occurring as the liquid nitrous oxide evaporates and takes up latent heat, but if the cylinder is switched off and allowed to rewarm the pressure will rise once more to that of the full cylinder as long as liquid is still present. Only when all the liquid is exhausted will the gauge pressure fall steadily to zero.
(A,R & L : p.174-176)

20 A C D
Caudal block is achieved by injecting local anaesthetic through the sacrococcygeal membrane into the extradural space in the sacral canal. The sacrococcygeal membrane covers the sacral hiatus, an opening caused by failure of the fusion of the 5th laminar arch. There is little likelihood of piercing the dura which normally ends at the lower border of S2. The average capacity of the sacral canal is 34 ml in males and 32 ml in females. It is a useful block for postoperative pain relief in children and the dose given is that generally recommended. The sympathetic outflow from the spinal cord ends at L2 whereas the sacral parasympathetic fibres leave with S2,3 & 4.
(A,R & L : p.44 & 770-774)

MCQ Exam 2 : Answers and Explanations

21 A C D
Theophylline is the pharmacologically active component of aminophylline, and by blocking the enzyme, phosphodiesterase, it allows the build up of cyclic AMP which leads to relaxation of bronchial smooth muscle. Salbutamol selectively stimulates the β_2-receptors in the lung and they in turn activate adenyl cyclase which increases cyclic AMP producing the same effect as above. Isoprenaline stimulates β_2-receptors as well as β_2-receptors in the heart, it therefore produces the same actions as salbutamol but in addition induces a tachycardia. Propranolol must not be given to asthmatics as it blocks the β_2-receptors in the lung. Aldosterone has no beneficial action in asthma.

22 B D E
Clonidine does act on α-adrenergic receptors but these are central in the hypothalamus and they are stimulated by the drug, leading to inhibition of the vasomotor centre. Trimetaphan acts on sympathetic ganglia. The other drugs are all peripheral α-adrenergic blockers, droperidol only weakly so, and phentolamine acting for a period of 10-15 minutes when given intravenously and phenoxybenzamine producing a prolonged block.

23 A B C D
D-tubocurarine has a weak ganglion blocking action which results in a fall in the peripheral resistance and a drop in systolic BP of up to 20%. Pancuronium causes a slight increase in peripheral resistance and a tachycardia, both of which are dose related. All nondepolarising muscle relaxants are potentiated by the aminoglycoside antibiotics, the effect is weak and is only seen clinically with very high doses. Being highly ionised muscle relaxants do not cross the placental barrier. Pancuronium is excreted in the urine and the bile, however prolonged action may occur in patients both with renal failure and with jaundice, so neither route can completely compensate for the absence of the other.

24 A C
Morphine stimulates histamine release and the secretion of catecholamines is increased due to stimulation of the adrenal medulla. Miosis occurs due to central stimulation of the pupillary fibres in the Edinger-Westphal nucleus and the impulse is carried in the oculomotor nerve, atropine can block the miosis. The sensitivity of the respiratory centre to changes in the arterial PCO_2 is diminished by morphine, but at normal therapeutic dosage the arterial PCO_2 is not usually much raised. The high incidence of nausea and vomiting seen with morphine results from stimulation of the medullary chemore-

MCQ Exam 2 : Answers and Explanations

ceptor trigger zone and not from direct stimulation of the vomiting centre, although this does become more sensitive to vestibular activity produced by body movement.
(A,R & L : p.108-112)

25   A B C D E
Chlorpromazine is a drug with many actions, and other phenothiazines with specific effects are usually more clinically useful. α-adrenergic blockade is prominent and causes peripheral vasodilatation and a fall in BP. Some phenothiazines can produce extrapyramidal effects that include Parkinsonian muscle tremors, if not recognised as drug induced they may cause confusion in diagnosis. Chlorpromazine has a marked anti-emetic effect which is due to a competitive action on the chemoreceptor trigger zone, but large doses probably also act directly on the vomiting centre. It has a mild anticholinergic, atropine like action, as well as being a weak antihistamine.
(V,S & W-S : p.78-84)

26   A B E
By definition this is the minimum alveolar concentration (MAC) of an anaesthetic agent required to produce lack of reflex response to skin incision in 50% of subjects. The MAC is unaffected by changes in the arterial PCO_2 or PO_2 over a wide range. It is affected by age; halothane has a MAC of 1.08% in infants and 0.64% at 81 years of age. Other inhalational anaesthetics reduce the MAC of any agent, the addition of 70% nitrous oxide reduces the MAC of halothane by about 60%. Narcotic analgesics lower MAC in a non-additive fashion. Premedication with 10 mg of morphine lowers the MAC of halothane by about 7%. The blood/gas partition coefficient does not influence MAC, but there is a relationship between lipid solubility and MAC.
(V,S & W-S : p.130-131)

27   A C D
Halothane produces a fall in BP proportional to the depth of anaesthesia and this is mainly due to direct myocardial depression. There are a number of other actions on the CVS which tend also to lower the BP, there is a central depression of the vasomotor centre and sympathetic ganglion blockade is produced. But the total peripheral resistance is unchanged at normocarbia, despite the obvious venous dilatation that is seen.
(S & A : p.135)

MCQ Exam 2 : Answers and Explanations

28 A B C E
Oxazepam is an active metabolite of diazepam as well as being available as a drug in its own right. Benzodiazepines in general are effective anticonvulsants and diazepam is of particular value in the management of status epilepticus. Chlormethiazole (Heminevrin) is a hypnotic with good anticonvulsant properties and has been employed for this purpose as an intravenous infusion, although it is more generally used for the symptoms of acute alcohol withdrawal. Thiopentone is also an anticonvulsant and has been used in status epilepticus, it is particularly recommended for convulsions occurring as a result of toxicity to local anaesthetics as it is likely to be immediately available in this situation.

29 A C
Propranolol, unlike practolol, blocks all β-receptors. Block of the β_1-receptors in the bronchioles may lead to bronchospasm and it is therefore contraindicated in asthmatics. In the heart the block of β_2 receptors reduces sympathetic drive and in paroxysmal nocturnal dyspnoea, a symptom of left sided cardiac failure, this may be dangerous. In atrial fibrillation, propranolol slows the ventricular rate but does not correct the dysrhythmia and although its use with digoxin requires care, there is no contraindication to the combination and in digoxin toxicity it may be specifically valuable when dysrhythmias are present. Changes in the serum potassium are relevant in digoxin administration but not with propranolol.
(V,S & W-S : p.385-387)

30 A
Cocaine is the exception amongst local anaesthetics in being a vasoconstrictor. Lignocaine and prilocaine have little effect on the vessels but the other local anaesthetics are vasodilators, hence the need to add vasoconstrictors such as adrenaline to them.
(V,S & W-S : p.212)

31 C E
Methohexitone is a barbiturate and as such is contraindicated in porphyria, dose for dose it is almost three times as potent as thiopentone. It is detoxified in the liver and excreted through the kidneys and gut. Excitatory muscle movements, tremor, coughing and hiccups are often seen but although methohexitone is contraindicated in epileptics as it can produce epileptic activity on the EEG, these movements are not themselves epileptic.
(A,R & L : p.255-256)

MCQ Exam 2 : Answers and Explanations

32   C D E
Chlorpropamide is a sulphonylurea and they act by stimulating the β islet cells of the pancreas to produce insulin. It has a half life of 24-40 hours and this may be even longer in the elderly; patients should stop taking it well before surgery. It is not metabolised but is excreted through the kidneys and it may be dangerous in patients with poor renal function. Alcohol intolerance occurs in about 30% of patients and they experience flushing of the face and neck, lightheadedness and wheezy respiration. Adverse effects are about twice as frequent as with tolbutamide, they include gastrointestinal upsets, rashes, vertigo, muscle weakness, headache, unpleasant taste, jaundice and blood disorders, but the latter are rare and are seldom serious.
(L : p.818)

33   E
Storage pressures in full cylinders are oxygen 1987 lbf/ sq in and nitrous oxide 638 lbf/sq in. There should be no water vapour in a nitrous oxide cylinder and storage at low temperature is not a problem, unlike Entonox which should not be stored below -8°C.
(S & A : p.224-225)

34   A B C D E
Dirt on the bobbin and static electricity may cause the bobbin to stick to the glass tubing resulting in large inaccuracies. Rotameters are calibrated for an individual gas at sea level, changes in the gas or ambient pressure will lead to inaccuracy. Ventilators that exert back pressure such as the Manley will depress the level of the bobbin and errors of up to 7% may result.
(A,R & L : p.149-150)

35   B E
The critical temperature is the temperature to which a gas must be cooled to be liquefied by pressure alone. A vapour can therefore be defined as a gas below its critical temperature. Liquid oxygen supplied to hospitals is stored in giant thermos flasks, correctly called Vacuum Insulated Evaporators (VIE). The pressure inside is around 1200 kPa and the temperature is about -165°C. As this is below the critical temperature of oxygen (-118.4°C) the high pressure turns the oxygen to liquid, at normal pressure oxygen would only be liquid below its boiling point, -182.5°C.
(H,H & T : p.19)

36   C D E
The saturated vapour pressure depends only upon the nature of the liquid and the temperature. At 20°C the SVP of halothane is 241

mmHg (32 kPa) and at atmospheric pressure, 760 mmHg (101 kPa), a mixture of air saturated with halothane contains 32% of the latter. At the boiling point the SVP is equal to the atmospheric pressure, thus if the atmospheric pressure is low as at altitude then boiling occurs at lower temperatures, hence the impossibility of cooking a hard boiled egg on top of Everest without a pressure cooker.
(H,H & T : p.77)

37 **A B C D**
Anatomically the three cervical sympathetic ganglia are fused with the upper thoracic ganglion to form the stellate ganglion. When they are blocked the sympathetic supply to the head and neck is lost. This results in Horner's syndrome : miosis, enophthalmos and ptosis. In addition there is dilatation of the conjunctival vessels, lack of sweating of the face on the same side as the block and nasal congestion (Guttmann's sign).
(A,R & L : p.675-676)

38 **B D E**
The ulnar nerve can be easily located in the groove behind the medial epicondyle of the humerus, it is best blocked 1-2 cm proximal to the groove to avoid the risk of neuritis. A successful block will produce sensory loss over the whole of the little finger as well as the medial side of the hand and ring finger. If the solution is sufficiently strong a motor block will also occur and the hypothenar muscles which act on the little finger will be paralysed. Although the ulnar nerve supplies the adductor of the thumb and on occasions the flexor as well, the remaining thenar muscles are supplied by the median nerve. Sensory supply to the ulnar side of the forearm comes from the medial cutaneous nerve of the forearm which arises from the medial cord of the brachial plexus.

39 **C E**
Carbon monoxide has an affinity for haemoglobin 210 times greater than oxygen and carboxyhaemoglobin is only slowly eliminated even in the presence of high oxygen concentrations. There is no effect on the chemoreceptors. Heavy smokers may have up to 15% carboxyhaemoglobin, which is one reason for the importance of stopping smoking prior to anaesthesia. The presence of carboxyhaemoglobin shifts the oxygen dissociation curve to the left.

40 **A C D**
The SA and AV nodes consist of rhythmically discharging cells, each impulse is followed by a declining membrane potential which triggers the next impulse, the speed of decline determines the rate of

MCQ Exam 2 : Answers and Explanations

discharge. Stimulation of the vagal fibres to the SA and AV node releases acetylcholine which slows the rate at which the membrane potential falls (repolarisation). The result is a decrease in heart rate and a prolongation of AV conduction.
(G : p.436)

41 None correct
The CSF is secreted by the choroid plexus in the lateral ventricles and passes through the 3rd and 4th ventricles to reach the surface of the brain. It is reabsorbed into the sagittal sinus by the arachnoid villi. It has a volume of about 125-135 ml and its pH and protein content are lower than the plasma being 7.23 compared with 7.35 and 24 compared with 40 mg/100ml respectively. The glucose content in CSF is 2.5-4 mmol/l compared with 4-5 mmol/l in plasma.
(G : p.489-490)

42 A B
Each litre of Hartmanns contains: sodium 131 mmol, potassium 5 mmol, calcium 2 mmol, chloride 111 mmol and lactate 29 mmol. A litre of normal saline contains sodium 150 mmol and chloride 150 mmol.

43 B C D E
Contraction of the diaphragm is responsible for 75% of normal inspiration but during expiration the diaphragm relaxes. The abdominal muscles are the most important muscles of active expiration, they act by increasing intra-abdominal pressure forcing the diaphragm up and also draw the lower ribs down and medially. The strap muscles are also involved in stabilising the thoracic inlet and larynx.

44 B C
The cerebral circulation, like the coronary, has insignificant sympathetic vasoconstrictor innervation and is therefore spared in the vasoconstriction that follows haemorrhage. Increased discharge from the baroreceptors inhibits the vasomotor centre and lowers BP, in haemorrhage therefore, baroreceptor discharge decreases.

Fall in BP and vasoconstriction in the renal circulation result in a fall in GFR. Production of both ADH and aldosterone increases causing retention of sodium and water.

45 A B C E
A rise in the venous filling pressure will increase the end diastolic volume and by Starling's law of the heart this will increase stroke

117

volume and cardiac output. On standing up from the lying position the venous return is reduced and the venous filling pressure falls. Increased body temperature and metabolic rate result in raised oxygen demand by the tissues and the cardiac output goes up to satisfy this. In the last trimester of pregnancy the needs of the placental circulation result in large increases in the cardiac output (approx. 1.5 l/min).
(G : p.456-458)

46 A
Changes in the arterial PCO_2 have a profound effect on the cerebral blood flow, at 8 kPa the rise would be about 50% above normal, whereas hyperventilation will lower the flow. A head down posture causes a rise in venous pressure and this decreases cerebral blood flow both by decreasing the effective perfusion pressure and by compressing the cerebral vessels. Autoregulation maintains a steady cerebral blood flow in spite of moderate changes in the BP. The effect of changes in PO_2 is small, a PO_2 of under 8 kPa (60 mmHg) will cause a slight rise in cerebral blood flow.
(G : p.495-496)

47 A B C
Whenever pressure is being measured with a fluid filled system, it is essential to ensure that the hydrostatic pressure of the fluid column is not altered by a change in the relative height of the patient and the measuring apparatus. This is particularly important when small pressures are being measured as with CVP. The position of a CVP catheter should always be checked with a chest X-ray as soon as possible after insertion, to ensure that the position of the tip is correct. Catheters can migrate into the right ventricle and if a sudden unexpected rise in the pressure occurs, this may have happened. Wetting of the cotton wool plug in the top of the manometer tube will delay or even prevent the fall in the fluid level and cause errors in the reading. Changes in the CVP resulting from straining during respiration and arterial hypotension are true physiological alterations.
(S & A : p.262-264)

48 D E
Pressures in the chambers of the heart vary especially in the atria, but in general normal values are: RA mean 1-2 mmHg, RV 28/0 mmHg, LA mean 5 mmHg, LV 125/3 mmHg. There should be no pressure gradient across the pulmonary valve, RV and PA systolic pressures should be the same, if the PA is lower then stenosis is present. Blood in the pulmonary artery is mixed venous blood having drained from

MCQ Exam 2 : Answers and Explanations

all the tissues of the body including the heart, it has a saturation of 75%. Having traversed the pulmonary circulation it arrives in the LA fully saturated.

49 C
Acetylcholine is the transmitter at ganglia in both the sympathetic and parasympathetic autonomic nervous systems. At the termination of the post-ganglionic sympathetic nerves noradrenaline is released, except for those in sweat glands which release acetylcholine. Acetylcholine is also released by post-ganglionic parasympathetic nerves.

50 B D E
The main hormone controlling sodium reabsorption in the kidney is aldosterone which acts on the distal convoluted tubule; ADH (vasopressin) controls water reabsorption in the collecting duct. The majority of sodium is reabsorbed in the proximal tubule by active transport, chloride passing out with the sodium. In the loop of Henle chloride is actively pumped out, sodium following passively. Starling's forces, the hydrostatic pressure and the colloid osmotic pressure, govern the movement of sodium, chloride and water into the peritubular capillaries.
(S & A : p.63-69)

51 B D E
Pyloric stenosis results in vomiting of acid gastric fluid alone, alkaline duodenal fluid being unable to pass the stenosis. There is hypovolaemia and a metabolic alkalosis resulting from the loss of hydrogen ions and chloride in the vomit. This leads to a characteristic pattern of the plasma electrolytes:

potassium	— very low
chloride	— low
sodium	— slightly low
bicarbonate	— high
urea	— high

The loss of chloride means that there is little in the glomerular filtrate in the kidneys, for sodium to be conserved something has to be exchanged for it in the tubules and at first this is potassium and results in hypokalaemia. As potassium becomes depleted hydrogen ions are exchanged, the urine becomes acidic and the metabolic alkalosis is made worse. These derangements in the kidney also interfere with the excretion of bicarbonate. Although metabolic acidosis stimulates the respiratory centre and leads to hyperventilation, a metabolic alkalosis

as is present here, does not seem to depress respiration to the same extent.
(V : p.333)

52 A B C E
The fact that blood groups are passed by Mendelian inheritance makes them of value legally in cases of disputed paternity. Approximately 75% of individuals are 'secretors' and have the same antigens as their ABO group in their body secretions, e.g. saliva, sweat and urine. Rhesus blood groups are independent of the ABO grouping and 15% of the population are Rhesus negative. AB blood cannot be given to other groups and although O negative blood is considered as universal donor blood, its administration always carries an increased risk when compared with fully grouped and cross-matched blood.

53 A C
Depression of the RST segment of the ECG is a characteristic change produced by digoxin even in normal dosage. Calcium gluconate is not of value in toxicity but if the serum potassium is low, the careful administration of potassium chloride either orally or intravenously may be beneficial but not if AV block is present. Phenytoin and lignocaine are quite effective in suppressing ventricular arrhythmias, phenytoin is also effective for the treatment of atrial arrhythmias. Corticosteroids are of no value.

Although plasma levels of digoxin can be measured, they are not a reliable guide as to the severity of toxicity as other factors such as electrolyte imbalance, age, thyroid disease and renal function will influence the severity of the toxicity.

54 B
Following transection of the spinal cord in man there is a period of about 3 weeks during which spinal shock occurs, all muscle tone is lost and there is flaccid paralysis. Muscle tone then returns but because all gamma efferent activity is lost, flexor tone exceeds extensor and the lower limbs flex. Shivering never occurs below the level of the lesion in spinal man. Micturition is a spinal reflex and is still present but the patient will have an automatic bladder. In the period of 14-28 days after the onset of paraplegia, suxamethonium administration may lead to dangerous rises in the serum potassium, but this is no longer a problem in longstanding paraplegia. Sweating is not lost, but can be markedly augmented as a result of uncontrolled sympathetic activity.

MCQ Exam 2 : Answers and Explanations

55 B D
In hyperkalaemia the P wave amplitude is reduced and the P waves may be absent. The PR interval may be increased leading to atrial standstill. The T waves become large and 'tented' and QRS duration is increased. Associated low serum sodium will accentuate these changes. Prominent U waves are seen in hypokalaemia.

56 E
In older men with prostatic enlargement postoperative urinary retention often occurs, drugs such as ephedrine and excessive fluid intake are well recognised as provoking factors. In women the problem is less common and perineal operations are the most frequent cause.

57 B C E
CPD blood contains few functioning platelets. The 2,3-diphosphoglycerate level remains normal for one week and then falls slowly. In stored blood potassium is released from the red cells and after 21 days the serum level has risen above 20 mmol/l, however some potassium is reabsorbed into the erythrocytes on warming and infusion. Anaerobic metabolism will raise the lactate level in stored blood and the breakdown of elderly erythrocytes raises the extracellular haemoglobin.
(A R & L : p.877)

58 None correct
Diffuse pulmonary emphysema leads to destruction of lung tissue but does not cause mediastinal shift or tracheal deviation. A right sided pneumothorax may result in deviation of the trachea to the left. Left pneumonectomy and left sided lung collapse can cause shift of the trachea but it will again be to the left. With nodal goitre, tracheal shift may occur to the opposite side.
(D : p.320)

59 B
A bronchitic who chronically had an arterial PCO_2 of 8.0 kPa (60 mmHg) would have a compensatory metabolic alkalosis bringing the pH back towards normal say to 7.35, with a base excess (BE) of say +6. In this case there has been no deterioration in the PO_2 or PCO_2 but his BE and standard bicarbonate (SBC) are normal. This must mean that there is an additional metabolic acidosis bringing his BE towards zero from what would be a 'normal' positive value for this patient. BE and SBC though very helpful in understanding acute changes can be difficult to interpret in chronic respiratory disease. Acute on chronic bronchitis would be characterised by a fall in pH with the BE and SBC staying the same.

MCQ Exam 2 : Answers and Explanations

A metabolic acidosis is normally characterised by a negative BE and low SBC but in these peculiar circumstances where metabolic acidosis develops against a background of chronic (compensatory) metabolic alkalosis, the BE and SBC are normal.

60 B C E

The normal response to a Valsalva has already been described (Paper 1, question 39) two types of abnormal response are seen.

1. A 'square wave' response occurs when the right sided filling pressure of the heart is high, as in congestive cardiac failure. The only change seen is a rise in the systolic pressure which lasts for the duration of the Valsalva. Because the right sided filling pressure is maintained, the other changes do not occur.

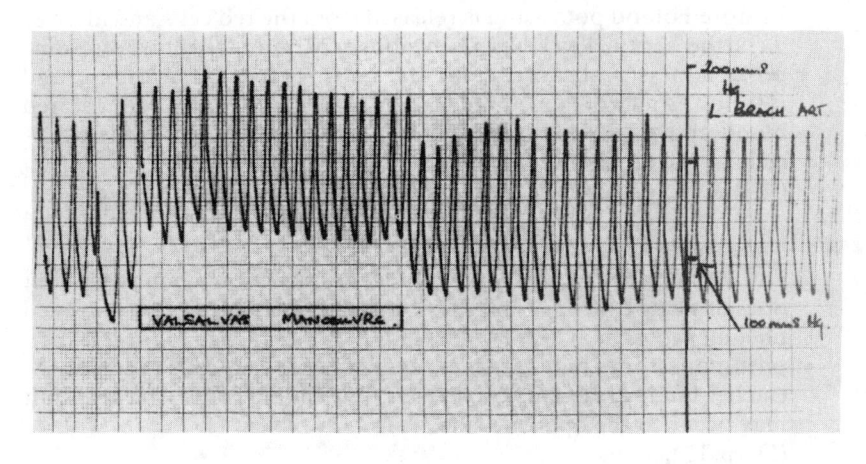

square wave response

2. A 'blocked' response seen when the autonomic nervous system is disabled as may happen with the use of adrenergic blocking drugs and in diabetic autonomic neuropathy. Here the initial response to the Valsalva is normal but the systolic pressure continues to fall as the subject cannot vasoconstrict. When the intrathoracic returns to nomal there is no overshoot in the systolic pressure which only gradually returns to normal.
    (S & A : p.46 & 47)

MCQ Exam 2 : Answers and Explanations

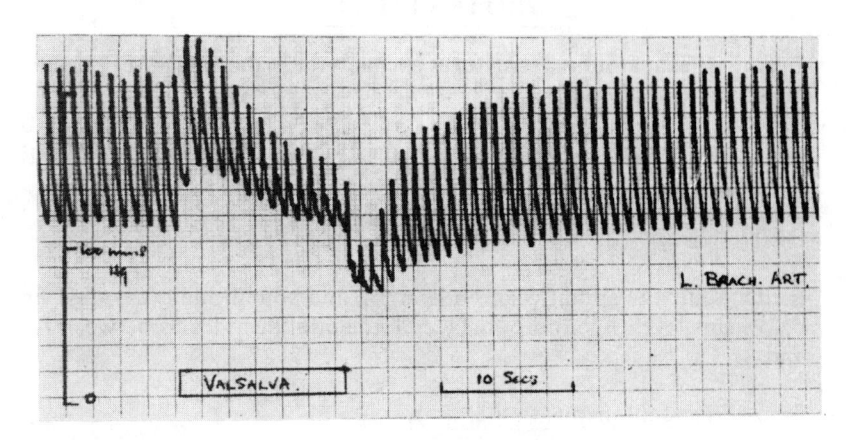

[Valsalva manoeuvre tracing — L. BRACH. ART., 100 mm Hg, 10 secs]

blocked response

THE WRITTEN PAPERS : OUTLINE ANSWERS

WRITTEN PAPER 1

1. **Describe the anatomical structures encountered in the passage of a needle for spinal anaesthesia.**

   A straightforward short anatomical question but details, particularly of the deeper layers must be thorough.

   OUTLINE

   In the adult the spinal cord ends at L2 and spinal puncture must be below this level. From the surface, in the midline at levels between L2 and S1.

   Skin and subcutaneous tissue.

   Supraspinous ligament, thick and tough, joining the tips of the spinous processes of the vertebrae.

   Interspinous ligament, thin layer between the spines.

   Ligamentum flavum, yellow elastic tissue, thick and tough particularly in the lumbar region, running from lamina above to that below.

   Extradural space, contains loose fat and plexus of veins, normally at negative pressure and really a potential space.

   Dura mater, strong fibrous layer with fibres running longitudinally.

   Subdural space, potential space between the dura and arachnoid maters, contains capillaries and lymphatics.

   Arachnoid mater, thin transparent sheath closely applied to dura.

   Subarachnoid space, contains CSF, nerves of the cauda equina and filum terminale (the continuation of the pial covering of the cord extending down through dura to the coccyx).

   If the needle passes on, it goes through the dural layers anteriorly and pierces the posterior longitudinal ligament before hitting the vertebral body.

2. **Describe the physiological effects of passive hyperventilation.**

   The question requires one to define the term passive hyperventilation and then describe the effects on various physiological systems.

OUTLINE

Definition: Ventilation of a patient to a lower arterial PCO_2 (normal 5.3 kPa). Passive implies the subject is not breathing spontaneously.

Effects:

1. Blood gases, PCO_2 decreased, pH raised, standard bicarbonate unchanged at first, PO_2 increased because of the lower PCO_2 (see ideal gas equation).
2. Renal compensation, increased excretion of bicarbonate bringing pH back towards normal (not reaching normal), standard bicarbonate falls.
3. Electrolytes, plasma potassium tends to fall as pH rises (potassium moves into cells to replace hydrogen ions), ionised calcium decreases (but total calcium rises slightly).
4. Respiratory centre, decrease or abolition of respiratory drive via central chemoreceptors.
5. Haemoglobin oxygen dissociation curve, shifted to left, decreasing O_2 available at tissues.
6. Neurones, increased excitability due to low ionised calcium: carpopedal spasm.
7. Cardiovascular, cardiac output decreases, vasoconstriction, uterine blood flow may fall, cerebral blood flow decreased with hypocapnia, ICP decreased, consciousness may be lost.

3. **A patient with chronic bronchitis is to have a general anaesthetic, what tests of respiratory function would be of value and what would be the significance of the results obtained?**

There are 2 parts to this question:

a) what tests
b) significance of the results

These are probably best dealt with together with a paragraph for each test.

OUTLINE

Introduction: Purpose of tests not diagnostic, but to assess severity, reversibility and progress of disease. Helps to decide on timing of anaesthesia, type of anaesthetic and seniority of anaesthetist. The simplest tests can be done at the bedside and can be repeated to assess preoperative treatment and postoperative progress.

Peak expiratory flow rate (PEFR) a simple bedside test, normal adult value 400 to 700 l/min.

Forced expiration (Vitalograph), FEV_1 and FVC but values obtained must be related to patient size and sex. FEV_1/FVC ratio normal value 70%, reduced in obstructive disease but in restrictive disease ratio unchanged or slightly increased because both values are reduced. Can be repeated after salbutamol to look for reversibility. If these are within normal limits one need not proceed to more complex tests.

Arterial blood gases, chronic bronchitics have a chronic respiratory acidosis, metabolic alkalosis and hypoxaemia. Estimation of pre-operative values will show if the patient is in best condition and will guide postoperative O_2 therapy and in severe cases the need for postoperative ventilation. Knowing the patient's 'normal' PCO_2 is important in reversal at the end of the operation.

Lung volumes, FRC, TLC and RV are all increased in emphysema which can co-exist with chronic bronchitis. If there is a large difference between FRC by helium dilution and thoracic gas volume by body plethysmography, this suggests areas of unventilated lung e.g. bullae, gas trapping.

Other specialised tests, carbon monoxide transfer factor and flow volume loops.

4. **What are the actions of intravenous barbiturates on the cardiovascular system? Discuss briefly their clinical significance.**

A fairly straightforward question in 2 parts. The word "briefly" in the second part indicates that more weight should be given to the first part.

OUTLINE

Thiopentone and methohexitone do not differ significantly in their cardiovascular effects, therefore consider them together.

CVS effects - vary with dose, speed of injection, bolus or infusion, age of patient and physical fitness.

Myocardial contractility	modest decrease
Systemic vascular resistance	little change
Venous capacitance	increased, blood pooling
Cardiac output	modest decrease
Blood pressure	modest decrease

Written Papers : Outline Answers

        Heart rate   increase
        Rhythm   no change

Local effects of intra-arterial injection of thiopentone - spasm, necrosis.

Anaphylactic or anaphylactoid reaction - rare, severe CVS collapse, usually previous sensitisation.

Clinical significance - normally effects are transient and are limited by the increase in heart rate but they can be much worse in those who cannot compensate, hypovolaemia, cardiac or adreno-cortical insufficiency, constrictive pericarditis, tight valvular stenosis, heart block. Administer cautiously. Effective in one arm-brain circulation time, therefore dose can be titrated to assess effect. Enquire for pain with thiopentone in case of intra-arterial injection.

5. **What are the indications for awake intubation in the adult? Describe the local anaesthetic technique that you would use for this procedure.**

Awake intubation is less often practiced in the UK than in the USA and indications will therefore vary according to local opinion, they can be listed briefly with the most relevant first. There are a number of alternatives for the local anaesthetic technique, for instance lignocaine spray can be used throughout but in an examination answer one should not make it too simple, the procedure below can be recommended.

OUTLINE

Indications (these are relative rather than absolute): the technique requires patient co-operation and full explanation
1. anatomically deformed upper airway particularly if sedation or anaesthesia may lead to loss of airway
2. immobile neck e.g. ankylosing spondylitis
3. inability to open mouth
4. respiratory failure requiring IPPV (to minimise use of drugs)
5. to avoid aspiration with a full stomach (as an alternative to cricoid pressure).

Local anaesthetic technique:

Upper airway, via nose 4-10% cocaine spray to both nostrils + 2% lignocaine spray to back of throat, or via mouth 60 mg amethocaine lozenge to suck, given 30 minutes beforehand.
Larynx above cords, superior laryngeal nerve which supplies the larynx above the cords can be blocked by the application of 8-10% cocaine to

Written Papers : Outline Answers

each pyriform fossa on a dental swab held in Krause's forceps. Larynx below the cords, (recurrent laryngeal nerve) crico-thyroid or trans-tracheal injection of 2-3 ml of 4% lignocaine during inspiration.

Absorption of local anaesthetic drugs from mucosal surfaces is rapid and maximum dosage levels must not be exceeded. If local anaesthesia is used with a full stomach the laryngeal reflexes should not be totally abolished.

6. **Describe your anaesthetic management of a 25 year old woman, who is 35 weeks pregnant and has developed appendicitis.**

An amalgamation of a standard emergency anaesthetic with the addition of the problems of late pregnancy.

OUTLINE

Preoperative visit, routine checks with particular reference to history of any problems during pregnancy, present condition particularly vomiting, past personal and family anaesthetic history, drugs, allergies; examine for dehydration and general fitness, check foetal heart; FBC and U&E's. Explain procedures, reassure, prescribe premedication as necessary. Give 30 ml of 0.3 Molar sodium citrate shortly before anaesthesia.

Induction, place patient on operating table with lateral tilt to prevent vena caval compression; set up IV infusion; check intubation equipment and suction, fully pre-oxygenate; induce anaesthesia with thiopentone apply cricoid pressure and then give suxamethonium; intubate, check tube placement.

Operation, maintain anaesthesia with usual anaesthetic drugs and relaxants (volatile agents which relax the uterus may be beneficial). Avoid maternal hyperventilation which may reduce placental blood flow; monitor ECG and BP and consider continuous monitoring of foetal heart.

Post-operation, ensure full reversal of relaxants, extubate in left lateral head down and keep on side until fully awake; give oxygen for at least 4 hours.

Local anaesthesia, for instance epidural anaesthesia could be used.

7. **Discuss the causes and treatment of a sudden rise in blood pressure during general anaesthesia for a laparotomy.**

Written Papers : Outline Answers

This is very much a practical question and it is important to show in your answer that you would look for common causes first and leave rarities to the end. Treatment depends very much on the cause so they should be dealt with together.

OUTLINE

1. Light anaesthesia, check nitrous oxide supply and vaporiser not empty, deepen anaesthesia with volatile agent or opiate.
2. Pre-existing hypertension, either undiagnosed or treatment stopped pre-operatively. Laryngoscopy is often the stimulus. IV β-blockers may be needed.
3. Hypercarbia, check breathing circuit and patient airway, CO_2 flowmeter not fully closed, with circle soda lime not exhausted, gas flows and ventilation adequate.
4. Hypoxia, importance of checking machine, checks as above, assess colour of fresh bleeding in wound and if necessary allow patient to breathe air.
5. Drugs, ketamine, cyclopropane, pancuronium, IV injection of vasopressor by surgeon.
6. Preoperative drugs, monoamine oxidase inhibitors interacting with opiates, clonidine rebound.
7. Fluid overload, stop infusion.
8. Hypoglycaemia, give dextrose.
9. Hormone secreting tumour, toxic goitre, phaeochromocytoma, carcinoid. Nitroprusside probably required.

WRITTEN PAPER 2

1. Describe the anatomical structures below the epiglottis seen during bronchoscopy.

The anatomy of the airway is asked about in a variety of ways, its anatomy and nerve supply should be known thoroughly.

OUTLINE

1. Laryngeal opening, lateral to the epiglottis on each side are the aryepiglottic folds containing the cuneiform and corniculate cartilages and posteriorly the arytenoid cartilages.
2. Enter the vestibule of the larynx which reaches down to the vestibular folds or false cords, pass through the gap between the rima vestibuli.
3. Enter the saccule of the larynx with the vocal cords below, thyroid

Written Papers : Outline Answers

cartilage in front and at the side, and the vocal process of the arytenoids behind, pass through the gap between the cords, the glottis (narrowest part of the airway in adults, in children the subglottic region is narrower).
4. Continue through the cricoid ring into the trachea with C-shaped cartilages lying anteriorly and laterally, after 10-12 cm in adults reach the carina.
5. Right side - main bronchus branches at 25° (distances from carina) 2.5 cm at 3 o'clock - upper lobe bronchus divides into 1. apical 2. anterior 3. posterior 4.0 cm at 12 o'clock - middle lobe bronchus divides into 4. medial 5. lateral 4.5 cm at 6 o'clock - lower lobe bronchus divides into 6. apical 7. medal (cardiac) 8. anterior 9. lateral 10. posterior.
6. Left side, main bronchus branches at 45°
5.5 cm at 9 o'clock - upper lobe bronchus divides into 1. apical 2. anterior 3. posterior + lingula 4. superior 5. inferior
5.0 cm at 3 o'clock - lower lobe bronchus divides into 6. apical 7. anterior 8. lateral 9. posterior (no medial on left).

2. **Describe the physiological mechanisms by which arterial hypoxaemia may occur.**

The logical way to tackle this question is by following the transfer of oxygen from the atmosphere to the mitochondria and noting how it may be diminished at each stage. This question only asks for arterial hypoxaemia so tissue hypoxaemia need not be considered.

OUTLINE

1. Breathing hypoxic mixture, high altitudes or unusual gas mixture.
2. Hypoventilation due to:
    respiratory centre depression
    spinal cord lesions
    anterior horn cells (polio)
    neuropathy (Guillain-Barre)
    neuromuscular (myasthenia)
    chest wall (crushed or flail chest)
    upper airway obstruction
3. Diffusion impairment e.g. interstitial fibrosis acting as a barrier to diffusion.
4. Shunt, blood reaching the arterial system without passing through ventilated lung, shunt may be:
    extrapulmonary (right to left shunts in the heart)
    intrapulmonary (consolidated pneumonic lobule)

shunts are the only cause of arterial hypoxaemia not improved by 100% oxygen.
5. Ventilation perfusion inequality, this is the main cause in many lung disorders (chronic bronchitis, pulmonary embolism).
6. Reduction of oxygen content in the blood (but not necessarily PaO_2 by anaemia, methaemoglobinaemia, carbon monoxide poisoning.

3. **Describe briefly the physical principles involved in the functioning of calibrated anaesthetic vaporisers.**

A short question but be sure to stick to the physical principles.

OUTLINE

1. Splitting ratio, the gas flow must be split precisely so that a set proportion passes through the vaporising chamber and the rest by-passes it.
2. Saturated vapour, gas passing through the vaporising chamber must be fully saturated with the anaesthetic agent, the chamber therefore contains wicks and baffles to ensure that the gas is fully saturated. The quantity of anaesthetic present will then be the saturated vapour pressure which depends only on temperature, at room temperature of 20°C this is known.
3. Latent heat of vaporisation, vaporisation requires heat and the remaining liquid will cool, this must be compensated for as the SVP falls with temperature and less anaesthetic agent is vaporised.

Methods:
   a. 'heat sink', vaporiser constructed of good heat conducting metal and having a large surface area.
   b. temperature compensation devices e.g. bimetallic valves.

4. **Compare and contrast the pharmacological effects of vecuronium and d-tubocurarine.**

The best way to compare and contrast is to take each aspect and discuss the effects of both drugs pointing out similarities and differences. You are only asked about pharmacological effects so history, manufacture, excretion etc. are not required.

OUTLINE

Both are non-depolarising neuromuscular blockers and show the characteristic pattern of fade and post-tetanic facilitation on peripheral nerve stimulation.

Potency, vecuronium 0.1 mg/kg approximately 5-6 times as potent as d-tubocurarine.

Onset, vecuronium faster than d-tubocurarine, intubating conditions in 1 to 2 minutes but over 3 minutes with d-tubocurarine, increasing the dose does not speed onset.

Duration, dose dependent but with equipotent doses vecuronium lasts 20-30 minutes and d-tubocurarine 30-40 minutes.

Potentiation, volatile anaesthetic agents especially enflurane, potentiate d-tubocurarine more than vecuronium.

Cumulation, with repeated doses, time and speed of recovery are not increased with vecuronium but they are with d-tubocurarine.

Recovery, once recovery beings, time from 25% to 75% of control twitch height is 11-12 minutes with vecuronium, longer with d-tubocurarine.

Reversal, both reversed by anticholinergics.

CVS effects, vecuronium devoid of CVS effects, d-tubocurarine decreases the BP by ganglion blockade.

Histamine release, none with vecuronium but occurs with d-tubocurarine and may cause bronchospasm in asthmatics.

Central effects, neither drug crosses the blood-brain or placental barriers.

5. **Describe in detail the management of intravenous regional anaesthesia (Bier's block) in the upper limb.**

   Preparation is as important as the technique.

   OUTLINE

   Preparation of patient, see the patient and check for contraindications — allergy to local anaesthetic drugs, sickle disease, Raynauds, scleroderma, severe neurological disease and possibly local infection. Explain the procedure to the patient, arrange for him to be starved and premedicate if necessary. Check equipment, full resuscitation equipment *immediately* to hand including method to administer oxygen by IPPV and to perform intubation, IV infusion equipment, drugs for

Written Papers : Outline Answers

convulsions, suction. Check the BP, have an open vein in other limb.

Technique

1. apply double cuff to arm
2. insert butterfly or cannula into distal vein (back of hand) and secure very firmly
3. exsanguinate the limb, if not painful Esmarch bandage or pneumatic exsanguinator, otherwise elevation for 3-5 minutes with occlusion of the brachial artery
4. inflate the upper cuff to 100 mmHg above systolic BP, note the time
5. inject prilocaine 0.5% plain solution, 3 mg/kg slowly
6. check the adequacy of the block

If necessary after 5 minutes the lower cuff may be inflated and then the upper cuff deflated. Cuff deflation, wait at least 20 minutes and if in doubt or patient is frail let down and re-inflate a number of times.

6. **A woman in shock is thought to have an ectopic pregnancy, describe briefly your anaesthetic management.**

Precisely the sort of situation that a Registrar at a DGH would be expected to deal with, as the exam is supposed to assess the candidate's ability for such a post, the written answer should be clear and to the point.

OUTLINE

Resuscitation must precede anaesthesia but this should be done quickly as only surgery can stop the bleeding. If BP low give oxygen. Initial assessment of blood loss, obtain good venous access, if shock is severe set up CVP and do blood gas to check for acidosis. Give IV fluid mainly colloid but also some crystalloid, FBC and cross-match 6 units and give blood when this is available. Look for filling of jugular veins, warming-up of periphery with filling of veins and pink colour, or CVP to satisfactory positive level. BP of over 100 mmHg if possible.

Premedication, should be minimal, atropine only; oxygen during transport to theatre.

Induction: ECG and BP recorder, induce on operating table if concerned; pre- oxygenation, cricoid pressure, whatever induction agent is chosen it must be administered cautiously, ketamine may be indicated in very shocked. Suxamethonium for intubation, theoretically relaxation of the abdominal muscles releases tamponade effect and causes more bleeding; surgeon should be scrubbed up and ready.

Maintenance: avoid all cardiac depressant drugs e.g. volatile anaesthetic agents at least until surgical control of haemorrhage, blood replacement intra-operatively (haematocrit 30%), fresh frozen plasma and calcium if tranfusion over 4 units.

Post-operation: extubate on side, head down, assess urine output and encourage if necessary, check haematocrit and continue oxygen.

7. **How may hypercarbia develop during anaesthesia, what clinical changes may result?**

There are a number of ways of approaching this question, one would be:

1. During spontaneous respiration
2. During IPPV
3. Others

Spend time to think of as many causes as possible. For clinical changes that result, go through the systems of the body, although most will be in the respiratory and cardiovascular systems.

OUTLINE

During spontaneous respiration:

Drugs depressing respiration, opiates in premedication or anaesthesia, barbiturates.

Deep anaesthesia, halothane for instance is a respiratory depressant and deep levels of anaesthesia lead to marked hypercarbia. Respiratory function, myasthenia, scoliosis.

Mechanical causes, airway obstruction, head down tilt especially in the obese, poor positioning e.g. prone, surgical retractors, assistants leaning on the chest.

Rebreathing, insufficient fresh gas flow for the circuit, increased dead space e.g. large mask on a small child, soda lime exhausted.

During IPPV:
Inadequate settings, ventilator set to insufficient minute volume for the patient, particularly likely with large patients or those with fever.

Leaks, in the ventilator or circuit. Dead space too large.

Others:
CO_2 administration, CO_2 flowmeter inadvertently switched on, CO_2 absorption when this gas is used for laparoscopy

Patient causes, increased CO_2 production e.g. fever, fitting.

Clinical changes:
CVS, increased catecholamine release, raises cardiac output, BP up, tachycardia, pulse full and bounding, local vasodilatation increasing bleeding, increased chance of arrhythmias especially with halothane.

RS, when possible increased respiratory drive leading to increased minute volume, respiratory acidosis moving the oxygen dissociation curve to the right.

CNS, cerebral blood flow increased leading to an increase in intracranial pressure, high concentrations of CO_2 have an anaesthetic action.

WRITTEN PAPER 3

1. **Describe the relations of the internal jugular vein, what are the common complications of internal jugular cannulation.**

   In anatomical questions, a diagram well labelled can save many words. Unless you are completely unable to draw this is recommended. The key word in the second half is common: at least 23 different complications have been described, you are not expected to list them all!

   OUTLINE

   Internal jugular vein is the continuation of the sigmoid sinus, runs from base of skull to join the subclavian behind sternal end of the clavicle forming brachiocephalic vein.

   Relations:

   Posteriorly: sympathetic chain, prevertebral fascia, muscles and transverse processes. At root of neck subclavian artery is deep to vein, as are phrenic, vagus nerves and dome of pleura. Thoracic duct on left.

Medial: lies in the carotid sheath with internal carotid artery anteromedial high up (IX, X, XI and XII between) and the common carotid and vagus medial lower down. Superficial: high up deep to parotid, lower down under cover of sternomastoid.

Complications:

Specific to this technique and related to the anatomy:
    carotid artery puncture (the commonest)
    pneumothorax (less risk with high approach and short needle)
    vertebral artery puncture
    nerve damage: Horner's (sympathetic plexus), phrenic, vagus
    thoracic duct (on left)

General complications:
    air embolism (importance of head down)
    haematoma
    sepsis
    thrombosis, thrombophlebitis

2. **Compare the physiological response to the infusion of 1 litre of normal saline with that resulting from the infusion of 1 litre of plasma.**

The sort of question that produces a chaotic answer if not carefully planned. The initial response is similar with both but the later effects are different.

OUTLINE

Both solutions enter the intravascular compartment which has a fluid volume of 3.5 l (plasma), normal saline contains 151 mmol of sodium and chloride and will slightly raise their plasma concentrations, the colloid content of plasma keeps it in this compartment, whereas normal saline will tend to pass out into the interstitial fluid which has a volume of 10.5 l and be held here by its sodium content.

Initial response: heart - increasing intravascular volume, CVP rises, stroke volume rises, cardiac output rises (risk of overload with rapid infusion leading to pulmonary oedema particularly with plasma).

Plasma osmolarity not altered therefore osmoreceptors not stimulated but increased volume stimulates low pressure receptors in atria, large veins and pulmonary vessels; ADH secretion reduced, more so with plasma.

Written Papers : Outline Answers

Later response: renal, increased renal blood flow and increased mean renal BP depress the renin, angiotensin mechanism and aldosterone secretion falls. GFR increased and with reduced aldosterone and ADH, urinary excretion of salt and water increased. With plasma infusion, the oncotic pressure will rise as water passes into the tubules and reabsorption of fluid is thereby increased.

Capillaries - with normal saline plasma osmotic pressure falls and reabsorption of fluid in the venous end of the capillary is reduced so that there is a net loss of fluid into the interstitial fluid; with plasma infusion the oncotic pressure is maintained and this does not happen.

Result: normal saline diffused into larger volume of interstitial fluid and also increased urinary output so that its effects are short lived; but plasma has remained in intravascular compartment and represents a very marked increase in its volume, therefore CVS changes maintained while level of plasma proteins is readjusted through decreased production.

3. **Describe the Mapleson classification for anaesthetic circuits indicating to which group the circuits in common use belong.**

A very straightforward question and one which you could probably answer in less than the allotted time by the use of diagrams. Once you have answered, use the time saved on another question. Further discussion of Mapleson circuits (e.g. of gas flows which was not asked) will not score extra marks in a close marking system. Remember to label the diagrams.

OUTLINE

Draw the systems which are in all the textbooks.

A. Magill attachment, Lack system is a coaxial version with expired gas flowing up the central tube.

B. & C. Only used in resuscitation or transport of patients.

D. The manual mode of many ventilators, Bain circuit is the coaxial version with fresh gas flowing up the centre.

E. Ayre's T piece for paediatrics, no bag.

F. Jackson Rees version of E with open bag at the end. (S & A : p.230)

4. **What is the safe maximum dose of the commonly used local anaesthetic drugs? What may occur clinically with overdosage.**

A short table will cover the first part but remember to give doses with and without adrenaline. The second part should be detailed but note you are not asked for the treatment.

OUTLINE

	plain	with adrenaline
Lignocaine	3 mg/kg	7 mg/kg
Bupivacaine	2 mg/kg	—
Prilocaine	5 mg/kg	8 mg/kg
Cinchocaine	1-2 mg/kg	
Cocaine (topical)	1.5 mg/kg	

Higher concentrations more toxic than weaker ones. Route of administration effects uptake and toxicity.

Overdosage

General signs: pallor particularly around mouth, nausea, sweating, yawning and drowsiness often precede true overdosage.

CNS: stimulation followed by depression; anxiousness, restlessness, hysterical behaviour, vertigo, tremor leading on in severe cases to convulsions and respiratory depression.

CVS: hypotension, bradycardia with feeble pulse leading to cardiac failure and arrest (with cocaine VF may occur without warning). RS: apnoea in severe cases due to central depression and respiratory muscle paralysis.

5. **Discuss the advantages and disadvantages of spinal and general anaesthesia for a patient requiring surgery for a fractured neck of femur.**

This is quite a topical question because of recent claims that spinal anaesthesia decreases mortality in patients with fractured hips. A good discussion is more than merely a list of pros and cons, it involves debate and argument. The outline below lists the points which should be covered.

OUTLINE

Make the general point: these patients are usually elderly and infirm.

Spinal: advantages, little effect on respiration, good for bad chest, decreased postoperative hypoxaemia, less risk of aspiration, some postoperative analgesia, reduced blood loss, decreased incidence of thrombo-embolism, minimises period without food and water, less problems with diabetics, some series show decreased early mortality but no difference at one year.

Disadvantages, takes a little longer than GA, difficulty of positioning a patient in pain both for block and on operating table, there is a failure rate, risk of fall in BP and need for vasopressors, nausea, vaso-vagal attack may occur in awake patient, patient may dislike being awake, frequent coughing in severe bronchitic, postoperative headache (use fine needle).

GA: advantages, quicker, no failure rate, hypotension (may be avoided by choice of technique). Disadvantages, greater incidence of postoperative chest complications and hypoxaemia, risks of full stomach in emergency case, more thrombo-emboli.

6. **Discuss the problems posed for the anaesthetist by patients with narcotic addiction.**

A complete answer is the result of bringing together many small points but stick to specific anaesthetic problems.

OUTLINE

Personality: often deceitful, difficult and aggressive, premedication may need to be heavy and include sedative agents

Venous access: nearly always a problem due to repeated thrombophlebitis and loss of veins, look at feet and legs or external jugular; if inhalational induction required second stage may be difficult.

Infection risk: abscesses, hepatitis, AIDs (wear gloves and take particular care to avoid pricking oneself).

Patient's general state: nutritional state often poor leading to risk of infection postoperatively, right sided infective endocarditis may occur, pulmonary disease due to septic pulmonary emboli leading to asthma and pulmonary oedema, unexpected hypotension may occur during anaesthesia. Withdrawal: cramps, vomiting and diarrhoea due to withdrawal may confuse clinical picture, difficult to know whether to treat symptoms or give narcotic.

Post-operation: analgesic requirements difficult to assess, tolerance to narcotics, patients may exaggerate pain or interfere with wound to get more narcotic.

7. **What action would you take when you find yourself unexpectedly, unable to intubate a patient at emergency Caesarean section.**

Every trainee should know a failed intubation drill in advance, this should therefore be easy to answer. Note the question says ' What action would you take': do not waste time discussing different strategies, choose one and give it. The other key words in the question are 'unexpectedly' and 'emergency'. A discourse on anticipating difficulty is not required. Emergency implies that waking the patient up and giving a regional block will be too slow, though this possibility should be mentioned. Tunstall's plan is the best known.

OUTLINE

Make the decision to abandon repeat attempts at intubation promptly.

1. Maintain cricoid pressure.
2. Place head down in left lateral position, get help from those around
3. Oxygenate by IPPV via face mask and oral airway, aspirate pharynx
4. If still obstructed try releasing cricoid pressure
5. If ventilation is easy establish anaesthesia with nitrous oxide, oxygen and ether by spontaneous ventilation. If you are unfamiliar with ether, halothane or enflurane can be used, local anaesthetic infiltration by the surgeon may also be given.
6. Pass stomach tube via mouth, aspirate, instill 20 ml 0.3 molar sodium citrate.
7. Level table, place patient supine with left lateral tilt and wedge, proceed with operation under spontaneous ventilation.

Additional points: if the patient is too light abandon attempts to pass the gastric tube, syntocinon can be infused if there is undue bleeding, pethidine can be given and halothane reduced after delivery, if unable to ventilate effectively allow mother to wake up, maternal mortality is more disastrous than perinatal mortality.

Reference: Tunstall, Anaesthesia 1976, vol. 31, p.850

ANSWERS TO THE CLINICAL CASE HISTORIES

Case History 1

Commentary

1. He is hypertensive, but a single reading should not be relied upon and he should be on a 4 hourly chart to see if his pressure settles.

2. The chest X-ray shows cardiac enlargement and unfolding of the aorta. The ECG shows left ventricular hypertrophy as evidenced by:
   a) tall R waves in V_4 (32 mm) and V_5 (22 mm).
   b) deep S waves in V_1 (14 mm), these can be confused with Q waves.
   c) S in V_1 and R in V_5 = 36 (greater than 35 mm)
   and left ventricular strain as evident by T wave inversion and ST depression in V_{4-6}.

3. The patient has serious hypertension which should be brought under control before he is anaesthetised, particularly for an elective procedure such as wisdom teeth. This operation should be postponed. There is now plenty of evidence that untreated hypertensives have higher anaesthetic morbidity than their treated counterparts.

4. This technique is not appropriate for a patient with cardiovascular disease. Cocaine, raised CO_2 and halothane all make ventricular ectopics more likely.

5. The fresh gas flow recommended by Bain for spontaneous breathing with a Bain circuit is 100 ml/kg and others have recommended higher flows than this. 6 l/min for an 80 kg man is certainly too low and is likely to result in hypercarbia.

6. Bigeminy: alternate beats are ventricular ectopics.

7. In addition to factors listed in 4 the surgical stimulus of dental extraction itself may cause arrhythmias. Halothane and raised CO_2 sensitise the myocardium to the effects of endogenous adrenaline which may be released if anaesthesia is light. The CO_2 may be raised because of the inadequate fresh gas flow with the Bain circuit. Partial obstruction will lead to a rising CO_2 and can occur during dental manipulation, movement of the head and the pack. Hypertension results if CO_2 is retained and may be particularly dangerous in this patient. Myocardial oxygen demand is increased while at the same time the increased ventricular wall tension may result in sub-

Case Histories : Answers and Explanations

endocardial ischaemia if there is coronary atheroma. All of which emphasise the fact that this patient should not have been anaesthetised until his hypertension was controlled.

Case History 2

Commentary

1. She has hyperosmolar diabetic coma, characterised by the high blood glucose and glycosuria with no ketones in the urine. The urea and electrolyte concentrations are raised because she is dehydrated. Serum albumin is raised for the same reason as are the haemoglobin and haematocrit (but see below). The leucocytosis suggests infection. The blood gases show a mild metabolic acidosis which would be consistent with her ill and dehydrated state. The acidosis would be much more severe if due to diabetic ketosis.

2. a) Osmolality = (2 x Na + 2 x K + glucose + urea) = 374 mmols/l (normal 290). The high osmolality draws water out of cells which is why the change in haematocrit is not a good guide to the amount of dehydration in these circumstances.

   b) Dehydration can be estimated by comparing the raised serum albumin (57 g/l) with an estimate of the albumin before illness, say 40 g/l. Then the fall in ECF volume = (1 − 40/57) = 30%. Her ECF volume would normally be about 15 l, so the deficit in ECF is 4.5 l and there is a further deficit in intracellular volume which is harder to estimate.

3. It is essential to correct the dehydration and metabolic chaos before embarking on anaesthesia and surgery. Diabetic gangrene is not an immediate life threatening emergency and the amputation can wait 24 hours which will be needed to correct the abnormalities.

4. 0.45% saline must be given to correct the dehydration and hypernatraemia. This must be done cautiously as too rapid a shift of water back into brain cells may exacerbate the cerebral state. Continuous insulin infusion will bring down the blood sugar and as this happens potassium will move into cells and potassium will have to be added to the infusion. Frequent electrolyte and glucose estimations are essential. (BMstix would be satisfactory.) CVP measurement will aid volume replacement. Broad spectrum antibiotics should be given to cover the infection. Once blood glucose is approaching normal the

Case Histories : Answers and Explanations

operative period can be covered by an infusion of 10% dextrose 500 ml 4 hourly with soluble insulin 10 units and 10 mmol KCl. The insulin can be increased or decreased according to blood sugar estimations. The regime should be continued postoperatively until she is taking food orally.

In choosing anaesthesia bear in mind that she also has angina, so cardiovascular stability is important. A unilateral spinal or light general anaesthesia based on a relaxant/nitrous oxide technique would fit the bill.

5. In these circumstances insulin would not be needed. Chlorpropamide is long acting and should be stopped for at least 48 hours preoperatively. It is better to change to the shorter acting glibenclamide a week or so beforehand. No drugs or breakfast on the morning of operation and provided blood sugar is less than 10 mmol/l hypoglycaemic agents can be restarted with the first postoperative meal. (S & A : p.488-491)

Case History 3

Commentary

1. The most striking abnormality is in the chest X-ray, this shows a large gastric shadow behind the heart containing air and a fluid level; the patient has a large hiatus hernia with most of the stomach being in the chest. The ECG shows lateral subendocardial ischaemia which might be expected in an obese patient. Biochemical results are in the normal range.

2. Arterial blood gases taken in the supine position, breathing air. This generally shows normal PCO_2 with decreased PO_2 due to a combination of factors producing increased venous admixture. A minority of obese patients have obesity-hypoventilation syndrome (Pickwickian) and have hypercapnia with somnolence, in addition to hypoxaemia.
Lung function tests. Rib cage movement is restricted and breathing is mainly diaphragmatic though the diaphragm may also be restricted by abdominal fat especially when lying down. This results in reduced Functional Residual Capacity (FRC) and Total Lung Capacity. Residual volume and closing capacity are unaltered so that closing capacity encroaches on FRC.
Urine and blood glucose (higher incidence of diabetes in obese patients).

3. 30 kg (43%). There are a variety of methods for estimating ideal weight one of the simplest is: ideal weight for male adult = (height in cm - 100 kg) and for a female (height in cm - 105 kg).

4. The general problems are: positioning and lifting the patient; it may be better to let him position himself on the table. Venous access may be difficult but it is essential for either general or regional anaesthesia. Intubation difficulties: one may need a detachable laryngoscope handle. Increased gastric residue of low pH with increased intra-abdominal pressure and risk of regurgitation. Cardiomegaly, increased work of the heart, increased O_2 consumption leading to subendocardial ischaemia. Those with hypoventilation syndrome may also have pulmonary hypertension, cor pulmonale and polycythaemia. Altered handling of drugs due to fatty infiltration of the liver and large mass of body fat with low blood flow; this will delay recovery from volatile agents. Variable absorption of IM drugs (more likely in fact to be SC), making post-operative analgesia difficult. Increased work of breathing with low FRC, making spontaneous ventilation inadvisable and incomplete reversal of neuromuscular blockade particularly dangerous. Postoperative hypoxaemia is exaggerated. Stress response to surgery will increase glucose intolerance.

5. The particular risk for this patient is posed by the hiatus hernia and high risk of pulmonary aspiration if precautions are not taken. The results of failing to take precautions are shown in Fig 6: aspiration.

6. Many of the problems above can be avoided by the use of regional anaesthesia but this can be difficult in the obese because land marks are obscured. Specially long needles may be required. Field block (iliohypogastric, ilioinguinal and genitofemoral nerves), spinal or epidural blockade would all be suitable.

If general anaesthesia is undertaken opiate premedication should be limited because of postoperative respiratory depression after a short operation. Benzodiazepines may be better. Pre-induction antacid (20 ml of 0.3 Molar sodium citrate) should be given. Rapid sequence ('crash') induction with application of cricoid pressure until a cuffed endotracheal tube is in position, can be followed by balanced anaesthesia. Atracurium has theoretical advantages for muscle relaxation because of its relatively short action and rapid elimination. Halothane is best avoided because halothane hepatitis is commoner in the obese. Enflurane or isoflurane will be more rapidly eliminated. Minimal monitoring includes ECG and BP. The patient should be extubated on the left side and not until the relaxant is fully reversed and laryngeal reflexes returned. Postoperatively ventilation should

Case Histories : Answers and Explanations

be checked particularly carefully, the patient sat up and oxygen given for 48 hours. Early mobilisation and heparin prophylaxis are needed for prevention of thrombo-embolism.

Case History 4

Commentary

1. The PEFR and FEV_1 are both reduced and FEV_1/VC is 56% (normal 80%). This is characteristic of an obstructive picture, i.e. typical of asthma. There is an improvement after salbutamol which shows the obstruction to be at least partly reversible. Vital Capacity (VC) is also reduced but less so than the FEV_1 and indicates some restrictive defect, though the asthma is clearly the main problem.

2. The first set of gases would be remarkably bad in an asthmatic if they were truly arterial. PCO_2 above normal in an asthmatic is usually the prelude to exhaustion and respiratory failure. The likeliest explanation is that it is a venous sample, these being normal venous gases. The femoral vein lies immediately medial to the femoral artery, which is not a good site for blood gas sampling. This explanation is confirmed by the radial sample which shows normal pH and PCO_2 and a mildly reduced PO_2 consistent with the patient's age and clinical condition.

3. Her hypertension seems reasonably controlled on Moduretic. One would want an ECG to look for any signs of left ventricular strain or enlargement. Moduretic is a mixture of amiloride and hydrochlorothiazide and is potassium conserving, but urea and electrolytes should be checked.

4. The two most important factors in choosing anaesthesia for this patient are to avoid provoking her asthma and to provide good relaxation for the repair of a large abdominal hernia. Epidural anaesthesia will accomplish this and avoid the need for intubation. Judging by the number of drugs she is on there is probably a considerable emotional component and there may be advantages in general anaesthesia. A relaxant, nitrous oxide, opiate anaesthetic with intubation and volatile agent supplementation would be acceptable, but it would be important to avoid histamine releasing drugs, most notably d- tubocurare. Many anaesthetists also avoid thiopentone in asthmatics as it is said to cause mild bronchoconstriction.

Case Histories : Answers and Explanations

5. Whether regional or general anaesthesia is chosen, good premedication is important. Standard anxiolytic and/or narcotic premedication may be given. Pethidine is frequently preferred in asthmatics because it relaxes bronchial smooth muscle. Steroid cover in the form of hydrocortisone 100 mg i.m. with premed must be given. It is also important to give salbutamol and beclamethasone inhalation with the premed or nebulised salbutamol via a face mask after premedication.

Case History 5

Commentary

1. The raised urea at the time of his admission is due to his being obstructed and it falls to within normal limits when the obstruction is relieved.

2. The ECG shows he has a pacemaker which is pacing on demand at 70/min. Note that where his own rate is greater than 70 there is no pacing spike.

3. Modern pacemakers are unaffected by diathermy. His particular pacemaker should be checked for this property. The diathermy plate should be positioned so that current does not go near the pacemaker (e.g. on the thigh). The pacemaker can be converted from demand to fixed rate by the application of a magnet, which should be available in theatre.

4. The fall in systolic pressure to 100 after the spinal is due to sympathetic blockade and is corrected by the infusion of Hartmann's solution. The fall that begins after an hour of operating could be due to blood loss, but the blood pressure is continuing to fall despite 2 units of blood and 500 ml of colloid. A likelier explanation is that large volumes of glycine from the irrigating fluid are leaking into the circulation (the 'TUR Syndrome'). It can be forced into open prostatic veins by the hydrostatic pressure of the irrigating fluid and can also leak if the capsule is ruptured. Both of these are more likely the longer the operation, and the more inexperienced the surgeon.

5. The diagnosis of fluid overload is confirmed by the investigations in recovery; dilutional hyponatraemia, pulmonary oedema and hypoxia with respiratory alkalosis. His confusion is due to a combination of water overload, hypotension and hypoxaemia.

Case Histories : Answers and Explanations

6. On examination the patient would be pale and peripherally cold, hypotensive with a raised JVP and possibly gallop rhythm. There would be fine crepitations over both lung fields. Fig 9 shows pulmonary oedema.

7. To Intensive Care. Diuretic therapy and IPPV must be started.

Case History 6

Commentary

1. Lung fields normal. Heart not enlarged. There is gas under the diaphragm.

2. Perforated duodenal ulcer.

3. Anaemic, with a microcytic, hypochromic picture suggestive of long standing iron deficiency anaemia. ECG essentially normal, sinus rhythm, rate 58/min.

4. Abnormal plasma cholinesterase: suxamethonium apnoea.
   Septicaemia.
   Anaphylactoid reaction to an anaesthetic drug.
   Malignant hyperpyrexia.
   Porphyria.
   Inappropriate dose of drugs, poorly managed anaesthetic.

5. Questions designed to distinguish between the above possibilites as well as the general question "Has anyone else in your family had a problem with anaesthesia".
   How long was the brother in ITU?
   Was he ventilated? For how long?
   Was he given any further instructions about future anaesthesia or drugs?
   Were measures taken to cool him?
   Patients are often surprisingly vague about family history and even their own past medical history. In limited time, one might end up not being able to exclude with certainty any of the three hereditary disorders mentioned above: abnormal cholinesterase, malignant hyperpyrexia and porphyria.

6. It might therefore be prudent to avoid barbiturates (precipitate porphyria), suxamethonium (apnoea) and all the drugs which may

precipitate malignant hyperpyrexia of which the most important are suxamethonium, volatile agents especially halothane, atropine, phenothiazines, lignocaine, curare. This does not leave much choice but, diazepam, etomidate, pancuronium, opiates, nitrous oxide (probably) could be used.
(AR & L : p.302, 527, 604).

In choosing the anaesthetic drugs one has to balance the risks: the probability of a full stomach and the possibility of some hereditary problem. One would take the usual precautions against aspiration (antacid, preoxygenation, cricoid pressure). The choice is then between using suxamethonium which undoubtedly gives the best intubating conditions or a nondepolarising relaxant which avoids any possibility of suxamethonium apnoea. For the inexperienced anaesthetist it may be better to use suxamethonium and test carefully for return of neuromuscular transmission with a nerve stimulator, accepting the fact that the patient might have to be ventilated postoperatively if he had abnormal plasma cholinesterase.

7. Despite the haemoglobin of 8.7 g this is clearly an emergency and one would transfuse the patient during rather than before the operation. Time should be allowed for cross matching (1-2 hours) but there need be no more delay than that. Chronically anaemic patients are usually well compensated for their low Hb, by increased cardiac output and increased 2,3-diphosphoglycerate (DPG) which shifts the oxygen dissociation curve to the right. Both of these factors increase oxygen availability in the tissues. Although transfused blood should increase the haemoglobin level and hence oxygen carrying capacity there may be disadvantages. Too rapid transfusion may lead to circulatory overload and congestive cardiac failure. Banked blood is low in 2,3-DPG which shifts the dissociation curve to the left and impedes oxygen release at the tissues. For these reasons transfusion immediately preoperatively (other than for volume replacement) is not recommended. One should not get too carried away with arguments about 2,3-DPG because within 6-24 hours of transfusion the levels are restored to normal. The main reason for transfusing this patient intraoperatively is because at a level of 8.7 he has much less haemoglobin in reserve to cope with expected and unexpected operative losses.
(V : p.336)
(S & A: p.501)

Case Histories : Answers and Explanations

Case History 7

Commentary

1. This is a normal chest X-ray.

2. The apnoea is due either to depression of central respiratory drive or peripheral neuromuscular failure.

    Central depression might be due to:

    a) Hypocarbia. A minute volume of 8 litres per minute for a 50 kg patient is well over 100 ml per kilo which might be expected to maintain normocarbia. A low carbon dioxide tension will reduce the central respiratory drive.

    b) Opiate depression. Fentanyl 200 mg in half an hour is generous on top of papaveretum 15 mg as premedication only an hour and a half before the end of the procedure at which point the papaveretum is probably exerting its peak effect.

    c) Other general anaesthetic agents, thiopentone and halothane, may contribute to central depression of respiration.

    Continuing neuromuscular blockade may be due to:

    a) Abnormal or low plasma cholinesterase causing prolonged paralysis with suxamethonium. The gene for abnormal cholinesterase is present in the homozygous form in approximately 1 in 3000 of the population. Such individuals take several hours to metabolise a single dose of suxamethonium.

    b) Failure to reverse the non-depolarising pancuronium blockade which might be encountered having used a high dose (more than 0.1 mg/kg) for a relatively quick procedure.

    A combination of the above factors can cause apnoea. Finally breath-holding on the endotracheal tube in a light patient may confuse the issue.

3. The clinical picture of a partially paralysed patient: twitching with uncoordinated attempts at muscle movement is quite different from the centrally depressed patient. A nerve stimulator should be used. Prolonged depolarising block (due to suxamethonium) will show diminished or absent twitch with no fade on tetanic stimulus. Non-

Case Histories : Answers and Explanations

depolarising block will be characterised by fade on tetanic stimulation or the train of four, and post tetanic facilitation. Opiate depression will be rapidly reversed by a test dose of 0.1-0.4 mg of naloxone. The respiratory stimulant doxapram (1 mg/kg) will usually reverse opiate and other central depression, but is nonspecific and does not help in diagnosis. Arterial PCO_2 will rise 3-4 mm per minute if the patient is apnoeic. If there is confusion as to whether the CO_2 has risen beyond normal and hypercapnia is causing apnoea an arterial blood gas should be drawn.

4. Patients with abnormal plasma cholinesterase need to be ventilated until the suxamethonium has worn off. The process can be speeded by giving fresh blood or plasma which contains significant amounts of the enzyme. Residual paralysis with pancuronium may be treated with a further dose of neostigmine, but remember that this will worsen a suxamethonium block. Central depression can be reversed with naloxone or doxapram as above.

Case History 8

Commentary

1. His lower mandible is somwhat receding but undue difficulty would not necessarily be anticipated.

2. Features which lead one to expect difficulty are muscular patients with short necks ('bull neck'), receding mandible, prominent upper teeth particularly if there are irregular gaps, limited mouth opening, limited neck movement, large tongue, obesity especially with large breasts. Tumours or trauma to the upper airway are obvious causes but often difficult intubation cannot be predicted from the patient's appearance.

3. Call for the help of a senior anaesthetist. At the level of Part I FFA you are expected to demonstrate safe rather than heroic management. (This is of course true at all levels of experience!)

4. Always consider: a) Wake the patient and do the procedure under regional anaesthesia. b) Can the operation be done without intubation either by controlled ventilation on a mask, or by spontaneous ventilation? The former is impractical in an eye case, but anaesthesia can be maintained by spontaneous breathing through a nasopharyngeal tube. c) Use more complex techniques to achieve intubation. In this case (a) was chosen.

Case Histories : Answers and Explanations

5. Although atracurium is of medium duration of action (20-30 mins), in common with other non-depolarising relaxants it can only be reversed with neostigmine when there is some recovery of neuromuscular function. A peripheral nerve stimulator will indicate this. Using the train of four, the fourth twitch disappears or reappears at 75% block and this can then be reversed with neostigmine 2.5-5 mg plus atropine 1.2-2.4 mg.

6. Surgical emphysema in the soft tissues of the neck, a result of trauma to the pharynx.

7.
    a) Passing a flexible gum elastic bougie (blind) and railroading a tube over it.

    b) Blind nasal intubation.

    c) Intubating the trachea with a fibreoptic bronchoscope and sliding a tube over it.

    d) Retrograde methods in which the cricothyroid membrane is pierced by a Touhy needle and an epidural catheter or Seldinger wire passed back through the cords to the mouth. This is then used to railroad a tube.

    e) Cricothyroid puncture and jet ventilation.

    f) Elective tracheostomy.

All of these techniques can be done awake with local anaesthesia or under general anaesthesia preferably with spontaneous breathing. b)- f) all require experience and should not be tried by the inexperienced solo anaesthetist. If there is doubt about the placement of the tube and cyanosis develops remember the golden rule "If in doubt - take it out" and ventilate by mask.

Case History 9

Commentary

1. No. All biochemical tests are normal and nothing in the history, such as weight loss, tremor, anxiety, tachycardia, suggests thyrotoxicosis. Patients with large goitres are usually euthyroid.

2. In hyperthyroidism T4 and/or T3 are raised and TSH is low due to

Case Histories : Answers and Explanations

suppression by the circulating thyroid hormones. In hypothyroidism T4 is low (T3 not usually measured) and TSH is high.

3. Lugol's iodine reduces the vascularity of the gland and is used to prepare the patient for surgery. The effect is only temporary and if the patient is not operated on within two weeks the gland escapes from control.

4. The chest X-ray shows the trachea deviated to the right by the enlarged thyroid.

5. Because of the deviated trachea a reinforced endotracheal tube such as the latex armoured tube should be used and a smaller size than usual may be necessary. The larynx itself should be easily visualised (the deviation being below this point) so no particular difficulty in intubation would be anticipated.

6. The pulse and blood pressure are both rising. The most likely explanation is that the patient is light or even paralysed but awake (euphemistically called 'awareness'). only 50 mg of pethidine was used for premedication, with atropine which would contribute to tachycardia. The technique of IPPV with 66% nitrous oxide, relaxant and pethidine supplement cannot guarantee that 'awareness' will not occur. Although this patient is receiving enflurane, 0.4% is a very low concentration and may well be inadequate.

    Hypercarbia is another possible explanation. Ventilation should be checked, but if the set gas flow (6 l/min) is being delivered to the patient who weighs 58 kg, this should be adequate.

    Thyroid crisis or storm is highly unlikely as an explanation because the patient has always been euthyroid and when it does occur, which is rarely, it tends to be later in the operation or during recovery.

7. If the right recurrent laryngeal nerve is damaged the right vocal cord will not move. If partially damaged the vocal fold moves towards the midline because the adductors are unopposed. If the nerve is severed completely the cord lies in the cadaveric (mid) position and in time the opposite cord compensates by increased adduction so that normal speech is restored.

8. Hypocalcaemia due to damage to or removal of parathyroid tissue. Tetany may occur, this can be provoked by tapping the facial nerve (Chvostek's sign) or inflating an arm tourniquet (Trousseau's sign).

Case Histories : Answers and Explanations

Calcium gluconate 10% up to 20 ml given by slow intravenous infusion will be needed.
(S & A : p.14. A, R & L : p.370-1)

Case History 10

Commentary

1. He has quite an extensive skull fracture over the right parietal area.

2. The positive Sickledex merely tells you that HbS is present. In the presence of a normal haemoglobin this is most likely to be Hb AS (trait). HBSS is always accompanied by significant anaemia. HBSC or HbSthal may be present without anaemia but these are rare.

3. Haemoglobin electrophoresis will give the definitive diagnosis, but this is not usually available out of hours. In this case a blood film should be examined for abnormal red cells and a reticulocyte count performed. The shortened red cell survival in HbSS leads to a reticulocytosis.

4. From the point of view of his head injury general anaesthesia, if it has to be given, should be designed to prevent rises in intracranial pressure and allow rapid recovery for postoperative neurological observations. This means ventilating the patient and avoiding halothane and enflurane. However, in this case a local block would be most suitable since it would not affect his cerebral state and would allow continued neurological assessment. Bier's block is contra-indicated (Sickle trait) but a brachial plexus block, axillary or supraclavicular, would be ideal.

Case History 11

Commentary

1. Sinus rhythm. Rate 75 per minute. Deep Q waves in V_{1-4}.
   ST segment elevated (Concave downwards) V_{1-3}.
   T wave invertion in I, aVL, V_{1-6}.

2. Anterior full thickness myocardial infarction. This is probably the reason for his admission to the hospital 6 weeks ago.

Case Histories : Answers and Explanations

3. Fitness for anaesthesia has to be judged relative to the urgency of the operation. The evidence is that recent myocardial infarction predisposes to a second infarct in the postoperative period. There is no doubt that his operation should be delayed because the risk of reinfarction falls as time passes, and medical treatment can be given as an alternative to surgery for duodenal ulceration.

4. To assess the risk in this patient one can only look at large series of similar patients. These show that the risk of reinfarction for surgery within 3 months of an infarct is about 40% and the mortality is higher (up to 50%). Between 3 and 6 months the risk falls to 15%, and after a year it is no higher than in other patients. Hence the strong recommendation to delay surgery.
(A,R & L : p.531)

Case History 12

Commentary

1. In a portable AP chest X-ray the plate is behind the patient and the rays are shot from anterior to posterior. In a PA film the plate is in front and the rays come from behind. The main difference is that since the heart is nearer the front of the chest it casts a bigger shadow in the AP than the PA view.

2. There is hyperinflation of the left lung with collapse of the right lung and a pneumothorax on the right. The collapse of the right lung is due to the endotracheal tube being down the left main bronchus (not clearly seen in this portable film). This would not cause the pneumothorax which may have been caused during insertion of the right internal jugular catheter which can be seen in all three films. The blood gases show marked hypoxia with normal pH and PCO_2. This is compatible with a large shunt which one expects with only one lung being ventilated.

3. The next film shows the endotracheal tube has been pulled back and is now in the trachea, but there is still a pneumothorax and the right lung remains collapsed. There would be no improvement in arterial blood gases.

4. A drain must be inserted with an underwater seal to drain air from the pneumothorax and re-expand the right lung.

5. The lung has re-expanded. The chest drain can be seen in the bottom

corner of the picture. ECG monitoring wires are seen across the lower chest.

Case History 13

Commentary

1. 2:1 heart block. The atrial rate is 84 per minute and the ventricular is 42. Only every second P wave is followed by a QRS complex.

2. Low cardiac output associated with this slow ventricular rate can cause dizziness, particularly if she changes from first degree heart block to second degree heart block (the rhythm shown here).

3. She should have a demand pacemaker inserted.

4. Certainly. If there is not time for the insertion of an internal pacemaker before surgery, temporary pacing with transvenous wires and an external box should be instituted.

READING AND REFERENCE BOOKS

ANAESTHETICS
Atkinson, R.S. Rushman, G.B. Lee, A.J. **Synopsis of Anaesthesia** 9th Edition 1982. Wright, P.S.G. (Abbreviation in text A,R & L)
Harrison, M.J. Healy, T.E.J. Thornton, J.A. **Aids to Anaesthesia, 1. Basic Sciences** 2nd Edition 1985. Churchill Livingstone. (Abbreviation in text H,H & T)
Smith, G. Atkenhead, A.R. **Textbook of Anaesthesia** 1st Edition 1984. Churchill Livingstone. (Abbreviation in text S & A)

MEDICINE
Macleod, J. **Davidson's Principles and Practice of Medicine** 19th Edition 1984. Churchill Livingstone. (Abbreviation in text D)
Vickers, M.D. **Medicine for Anaesthetists** 2nd Edition 1982. Blackwell. (Abbreviation in text V)

PHYSIOLOGY
Ganong, W.F. **Review of Medical Physiology** 11th Edition 1985. Lange. (Abbreviation in text G)

PHARMACOLOGY
Laurence, D.S. Bennet, P.N. **Clinical Pharmacology** 5th Edition 1984. Churchill Livingstone. (Abbreviation in text L)
Vickers, M.D. Schneiden, H. Wood-Smith, F.G. **Drugs in Anaesthetic Practice** 6th Edition 1980. Butterworths. (Abbreviation in text V, S & W-S)

ACKNOWLEDGEMENTS

We are grateful to the following for permission to reproduce certain diagrams.

Diagram p.98. Campbell, Dickenson and Slater. Clinical Physiology. 3rd edition 1968. Blackwell Scientific.

Diagram p. 101. Wood. Diseases of the Heart. 1956 Lippincott.

Diagrams p. 122, 123. Churchill-Davidson. A Practice of Anaesthesia. 4th edition 1979. Lloyd Luke Ltd.

INDEX

Only the key words in the question sections have been included in this index, its purpose being to enable questions on particular topics to be found:

adrenal cortex, hormones 21
α-adrenergic receptors 29
albumin 18
angina pectoris 22, 48
anticonvulsant drugs 30
apnoea, postoperative 55
appendicitis 41
arrhythmias 12
asthma 29, 50
atropine 16
autonomic ganglia, transmitters 36

barbiturates, intravenous 41
blood
    gases 21, 25, 38, 48, 51, 52, 61
    glucose 14
    groups 36
    loss 34
    stored 38
    warming 26
blood pressure 17
    sudden rise 41
Boyles machine 26
brachial plexus block,
    supraclavicular 11
bronchitis, chronic 22, 23, 38, 41
bronchoscopy, anatomy 42
bupivacaine 16

carbon dioxide, transport 19
carbon monoxide 33
cardiac output 35
caudal block 28
central venous pressure 20, 35
cerebral blood flow 35
cerebrospinal fluid 34
cervical sympathetic ganglia,
    block 33
chlorpromazine 30
chlorpropamide 31
clonidine 10
convulsions 11

critical pressure 17
critical temperature 32
cylinders 32

dantrolene 15
dextran infusion 27
diabetes mellitus 48
digoxin 14
    toxicity 37
dissociation curve 19
divers 17
dopamine 14
drug dependence 16
drugs, induction 10
d-tubocurarine 42

ECG 22, 60, 62
hyperkalaemia 37
emphysema 23
enflurane 9
epigastric pain 54
ethers, halogenated 25
expiration 34
explosive anaesthetics 13

familial problems 54
fat embolism 27
first rib 18
functional residual capacity 21

gallstones 23
glycine 22
Guedel's classification 28

halothane 9, 13, 24, 30
Hartmann's solution 34
head injury 59
heart
    block 62
    normal 20, 35
helium 17
high altitude 20

157

Index

hip fracture 12, 43
hiatus hernia 49
hyoscine 16
hypercarbia 42
hypertension 10
  untreated 47
hyperventilation, passive 41
hypoxaemia 42

intravenous
  infusion 43
  injection, pain 26
  regional anaesthesia 9, 42
intubation
  awake 41
  difficult 43, 56
  right main bronchus 24
isoflurane 15

ketamine 14
knee jerk 19

laminar flow 17
lignocaine, overdosage 25
local anaesthetic drugs,
    overdosage 43

MAC 13, 30
Magill circuit 11
malignant hyperpyrexia 13, 24
Mapleson classification 43
methohexitone 31
minute volume 19
morphine 29
myocardial infarction 60

naloxone 15
narcotic addiction 43
neuromuscular block 11
  depolarising 16, 24
  non-depolarising 27
nitrous oxide 28
nodal rhythm 13

obesity 26, 49
oxygen 28

pacemaker 52
pancuronium 29
pathology results 12
pneumothorax 61
potassium 23, 27
pregnancy 41
  ectopic 42
propranolol 31
pulmonary function tests 50
pyloric stenosis 36

Raynaud's phenomenon 21
renal function, normal 20
respiratory depression 15
respiratory function tests 41
rotameter 32

saturated vapour pressure 32
sickle cell disease 23, 59
soda lime 9
sodium 23
  reabsorption 36
spinal anaesthesia, anatomy 41
spinal cord, transection 37
suxamethonium 16

thiopentone 10, 15
thrombosis 10
thyroidectomy 57
tourniquet 12
trachea, shift 38
trichlorethylene 25
TURP 22, 52

ulnar nerve, block 33
urinary retention,
    postoperative 37
uterine tone 9

vagus 33
Valsalva manoeuvre 18, 38
vaporiser 10, 42
vasoconstriction 31
vecuronium 42
vein
  basilic 18
  internal jugular 43